PATHWAYS TO A SUCCESSFUL
ACCOUNTABLE CARE ORGANIZATION

PATHWAYS TO A SUCCESSFUL ACCOUNTABLE CARE ORGANIZATION

Edited by PETER A. GROSS, MD

JOHNS HOPKINS UNIVERSITY PRESS | *Baltimore*

This book was brought to publication with the generous support of the David E. Ryer Director's Endowment and the Robert L. Warren Endowment.

Johns Hopkins University Press
2715 North Charles Street
Baltimore, Maryland 21218-4363
www.press.jhu.edu

Library of Congress Cataloging-in-Publication Data

Names: Gross, Peter A., 1938–2020 editor.
Title: Pathways to a successful accountable care organization / edited by
    Peter A. Gross, MD.
Description: Baltimore : Johns Hopkins University Press, 2020. |
    Includes bibliographical references and index.
Identifiers: LCCN 2019040490 | ISBN 9781421438252 (paperback ; alk. paper) |
    ISBN 9781421438269 (ebook)
Subjects: MESH: Accountable Care Organizations | Quality Assurance,
    Health Care—methods | Primary Health Care—trends
Classification: LCC RA425 | NLM W 84.41 | DDC 362.1—dc23
LC record available at https://lccn.loc.gov/2019040490

A catalog record for this book is available from the British Library.

*Special discounts are available for bulk purchases of this book. For more
information, please contact Special Sales at specialsales@press.jhu.edu.*

CONTENTS

JOSHUA BENNETT, MD, MBA, Independent Clinical Consultant and
Physician Reviewer, National Committee for Quality Assurance
on ACOs and Patient-Centered Medical Homes, Washington, DC.
Formerly Principal, Premier Inc., Charlotte, NC.

GLEN CHAMPLIN, Principal, Premier Inc., Charlotte, NC.

KRIS CORWIN, JD, MHA, Former Senior Project Manager, Discern
Health, Baltimore, MD. He previously worked at the National
Committee for Quality Assurance and the Leapfrog Group.

GUY D'ANDREA, Managing Partner, Discern Health, Baltimore, MD.

JOSEPH F. DAMORE, FACHE, Service Line Vice President of Strategy,
Innovation, and Population Health, Premier Inc., Charlotte, NC.

MITCHEL EASTON, ACO Data Analytics Manager, Hackensack
Alliance ACO, Hackensack, NJ.

ANDY EDEBURN, MA, Principal, Population Health, Premier Inc.,
Charlotte, NC, and Minneapolis, MN.

SETH EDWARDS, MHA, Vice President of Population Health
Management, Premier Inc., Charlotte, NC. He leads Premier's
Population Health Management Collaborative comprising more
than 75 health systems and clinically integrated networks. Seth
was named a *Modern Healthcare* Up & Comer in 2018.

KRIS GATES, JD, CEO, Health Endeavors, Scottsdale, AZ. She
developed the ACO quality measure tracking and reporting
technology used by more than 90 Medicare ACOs and is author
of the book *One Touch Health "Smart Record."*

SHAWN GRIFFIN, MD, President and CEO, URAC, Washington, DC.
Formerly Chief Quality and Informatics Officer, Memorial
Hermann Physician Network (MHMD).

Peter A. Gross, MD, Chairman, Hackensack Alliance ACO, Hackensack, NJ. Formerly Executive Vice President and Chief Medical Officer, Hackensack University Medical Center. Former NAACOS Board Member. Professor of Medicine, Hackensack Meridian School of Medicine at Seton Hall University.

Brent Hardaway, MS, President, R. B. Hardaway Consulting LLC, Austin, TX. Formerly Vice President of Population Health Advisory Services, Premier Inc.

Mark Hiller, MBA, Vice President of Bundled Payment Services, Premier Inc., Charlotte, NC.

Beth Ireton, RN, MS, Principal, Premier Inc., Charlotte, NC.

Thomas Kloos, MD, President of Atlantic ACO, Morristown, NJ, and Management Services Organization Director for Optimus ACO, Summit, NJ. Current member of the National Association of ACOs Board of Directors.

Jeremy Mathis, MBA, Lean Cert., Director, Population Health Management, Premier Inc., Charlotte, NC.

Miriam McKisic, Manager, Performance Partner, Premier Inc., Charlotte, NC.

Morey Menacker, DO, President and CEO of Hackensack Alliance ACO 2012–2018, Hackensack, NJ.

Denise Patriaco, RN, APN-C, Administrative Director, Hackensack Alliance ACO, Hackensack, NJ, and Regional Director for Population Health, North Region of Hackensack Meridian Health System.

Elyse Pegler, MPH, Principal, Population Health, Premier Inc., Charlotte, NC.

John Pitsikoulis, Principal, Premier Inc., Charlotte, NC.

Michael Schweitzer, MD, MBA, Chief of Population Health, Verity Health System, Redwood City, CA.

Bryan F. Smith, MS, Principal, Economic and Analytic Advisory Services, Population Health Management, Premier Inc., Charlotte, NC.

Overview

Health care in America is undergoing great change. The fee-for-service approach to paying for medical services is doomed. The Centers for Medicare and Medicaid Services (CMS) is orchestrating a fundamental change from an emphasis on the volume of health care services to a more logical and necessary emphasis on generating value for those same services. To assess the value of services, quality metrics have been developed that determine the merit of the patient experience, the ability to improve the health of a population, and how providers can reduce the cost of care. This is known as the Triple Aim, or stated briefly: better care, better health, at lower cost. To accomplish the Triple Aim, CMS has created at least three alternatives that are being tested simultaneously in the real world of health care: accountable care organizations (ACOs), Bundled Payment for Care Improvement (BPCI), and the Merit-based Incentive Payment System (MIPS) that was borne out of the Medicare Access and CHIP Reauthorization Act of 2015. Tens of millions of people are already part of these three experimental changes. Soon it will include most providers in the United States. Our book describes how these three improvement approaches for health care facilitate attaining the Triple Aim. Going forward, businesses and health care systems have a choice—to be either a catalyst for change by heeding the recommendations in our book or a casualty of the change.

Over 1,000 ACOs have been created in the United States. Approximately half were formed with CMS. The emphasis in our book is on CMS's ACOs, though we also include a detailed description of BPCI and MIPS. CMS adds approximately 100 ACOs every year. Their program is known as the Medicare Shared Savings Program, in which CMS and the

ACO split 50/50 the savings that exceed a certain level. The split occurs only when compliance with the numerous quality measures is sufficient. Originally, most ACOs signed on to share upside financial gains only, with no sharing of losses. Sharing losses is referred to as "downside risk." Now, after six years, CMS is changing the rules such that all programs will eventually have to be responsible for losses—downside risk—when they don't generate upside savings, or gains. CMS feels that savings will be more likely to occur when the providers in ACOs are responsible for downside risk. This proposed rule change was announced in August 2018. The final rule, issued in December 2018, confirmed this change. Our chapters include the necessary components of the final rule.

Let's review here how we got into this position.

Evolution of Medicine

Starting with the Father of Western Medicine, Hippocrates of Kos (460–377 BC) from the Classical Age of Greece, the basis of medicine moved from supernatural ideas about cause and cure of illnesses to the natural theory of disease. This change was further supported by Galen of Pergamon (129–210 AD) who identified arteries as the carrier of blood. Then William Harvey (1578–1657) discovered the complete path for blood circulation.

Edward Jenner (1746–1823), with his work on cowpox prevention, became the first person to describe the benefits of vaccination, in particular smallpox vaccine. Now the disease has been eradicated due to a successful worldwide vaccination campaign. Joseph Lister (1827–1912) pioneered the use of sterile technique in surgical procedures. The further development of the Jenner's and Lister's discoveries became the basis of additional improvements in health care. Their findings fostered the widespread application of vaccination for many different diseases and the application of public health polices geared to improving the hygiene of populations.

Further understanding of the causes of infectious diseases, the primary killers at that time, was generated by several key figures. The Frenchman Louis Pasteur (1822–1895) demonstrated the benefits of pasteurization. The German Robert Koch (1848–1910) identified the causes of tuberculosis, cholera, and anthrax, among the deadliest of human and animal diseases. The Czech psychoanalyst Sigmund Freud (1856–1939) gave us an inside look at human behavior and its effect on our health. The discoveries of Scotsman Alexander Fleming (1881–1955) moved us to the next stage of conquering bacterial infectious diseases with his discovery of penicillin. The American Jonas Salk (1914–1995) eliminated the viral epidemic of polio, the scourge of the early and mid-twentieth century. The space created by the amelioration of infectious diseases became filled by a relative increase in cardiac diseases and cancer, the next phase in our effort to reduce the impact of all diseases on populations.

Evolution of Payment Mechanisms

The march of science has prolonged life. But how do we pay for these amazing advances? As medical and surgical treatments became more common and more expensive, paying for them was a major issue. The occurrence of these diseases became a particular financial burden on the older population. In 1965, President Lyndon Johnson created Medicare and Medicaid to provide financial support for the older population and the infirmed. These services continued to be increasingly expensive. Fee-for-service was how the doctor and hospital bills were paid. To try to reduce these expenses, health maintenance organizations (HMOs) were started in 1974, based in part on a model at the Marshfield Clinic in Wisconsin. Insurers, however, encouraged the sick to go to the Marshfield Clinic and healthy patients to go elsewhere. This selfish approach led to the clinic's failure. Nevertheless, HMOs spread across the United States with the help of the federal HMO Act of 1973. It was a prepaid capitated system that replaced fee-for-service. Over the years, it assumed many different forms of payment and care. In the 1990s, patients started complaining about services denied and referrals refused. Eventually, preferred provider organizations (PPOs) replaced HMOs. PPOs were just discounted fee-for-service organizations. There was no incentive to organize integrated delivery systems or improve the quality of care. In 1983, diagnosis-related groups were added to standardize the prospective payment system, but they only applied to hospital payments and not to physician payments. The goal was to encourage cost containment in hospitals by providing payment targets for specific diagnoses instead of paying for hospital length of stay. But it did not deal effectively with reducing the rapidly rising costs of care or address the issue of care quality.

Evolution of Quality Measurement

The quality issues in health care began to be recognized in the later nineteenth and early twentieth centuries. Some of the early pioneers were the American Ernest Codman (1869–1940) in medicine and the Italian Florence Nightingale (1820–1910) in nursing. Codman advocated for the "end result," namely, that you should follow the surgical patient long enough after surgery to determine if the surgical procedure was successful, and if not, why. While in his time his approach was not greeted with enthusiasm, his ideas and findings ultimately led to the creation of the Joint Commission on Accreditation of Hospitals, today known as The Joint Commission. Nightingale developed her ideas after seeing the abysmal care during a cholera outbreak among British troops in the Crimea War (1853–1856). She implemented many practices taken for granted today:

a. Infection control to keep her facility clean
b. Requirements for patients to care for themselves, if they could, to promote healing
c. Rounding on hospital beds at night with a lamp (hence, "the lady with the lamp") to check patient progress
d. Emphasized therapeutic communication during rounds in order to initiate empathic discussions with patients
e. Offering spiritual nursing for comfort in a patient's final days

It soon became apparent that to improve quality, it had to be measured. Avedis Donabedian (1919–2000) developed the construct to do just that. His system for measuring quality was to identify three types of quality measures: structural, process, and outcome. He said that structural measures affect process measures, which in turn affect outcome measures. For example, many outcome measures are called process-oriented outcome measures. To identify unintended consequences of following one of these measures, he introduced the concept of the balancing measure.

Today one of the chief proponents of measuring quality of care is Donald Berwick (1946–present). He introduced the concept of the Triple Aim. Berwick was president of the Institute for Healthcare Improvement as well as the former administrator of CMS at the time when the ACO concept was being promoted to practicing physicians and hospitals. The Triple Aim's formal goals are to

1. improve the experience of care,
2. improve the health of populations, and
3. reduce per capita costs of health care.

Improving quality usually costs less, not more, because it eliminates wasteful practices.

Another key component for improving care quality is to coordinate the care itself. Coordination should be the shared responsibility of the physicians, the nurses, and the health care setting, such as the hospital. Since the turn of the last century, it's almost always been nurses who have carried out this major task. Now under the ACO concept, care coordination has received renewed emphasis in which all parties must be involved equally, and measures have been created to monitor whether coordination is actually happening.

To assist physicians in developing and applying a program to coordinate care and to systematically and consistently apply quality improvement principles to all of their patients, the National Committee for Quality Assurance (NCQA) was created in 1990. It developed the patient-centered medical home (PCMH) program, which transforms the physician's office practice into a higher quality, patient-focused coordinated care provider. The PCMH program emphasizes patient access and appointment availability, care management, and care transformation. It provides regular performance results, assures the rights of patients, and identifies the responsibilities of the providers. If properly implemented, the practice can achieve "recognition" from NCQA or two other organizations.

As you can imagine, many quality measures have been written, and selecting which ones to use is often problematic. To help solve this dilemma, the National Quality Forum (NQF) was created in 1999. NQF is the final arbiter on the validity of implementing a specific measure. Its goal is to identify measures that improve patient health, enhance quality, and help manage costs. Its criteria for certifying a quality measure are

Is the measure scientifically valid and replicable?
Is the measure feasible in real-world health care?
Will it be useful to and used by providers and patients?
Will the measure add value to existing measurement and improvement efforts?

The next issue is what to do with all this information on quality. Data analytic software was created to assist in the collection of quality and cost information. It is available to assess performance. Some of the clinical areas where such software is used are the frequency of hospital admissions, readmissions, emergency room stays, and skilled nursing facility visits. This administrative data can be viewed by the health care system, hospital, practice, or individual provider. With the availability of electronic health records, clinical data, such as compliance with quality measures, can also be viewed by the health care system, hospital, practice, or individuals. The quality measures themselves can address deficiencies in the application of preventive vaccines (e.g., influenza and pneumococcal vaccines), early detection of cancer procedures (e.g., colonoscopy, mammography), tests for disease control (e.g., hemoglobin A1c), and patient experiences using the Consumer Assessment of Healthcare Providers and Systems.

To be fair in the assessment of the quality of care, assessors need to be aware of a variety of determinants of health as they may influence, for example, the degree of patient compliance with a physician recommendation to test for hemoglobin A1c, to have a colonoscopy performed, or to receive influenza vaccine. The determinants influence the proportion in or out of compliance with recommendations. Examples of the determinants include:

- Biologic or genetic: presence of a cystic fibrosis gene in a parent or existence of lymphoma in a patient
- Social: presence of lower socioeconomic circumstances or education level
- Behavioral: presence of physical inactivity, a smoking habit, or mental illness
- Environmental: exposure to poor sanitation, risky occupational conditions, or atmospheric pollution
- Health care: presence of quality and access to care, use of antihypertensive medications

Ironically, appropriate health care accounts for only 10% of the social determinant's effect on good health. The poor often have a combination of inadequate social circumstances, abnormal behavioral patterns, and adverse environmental exposure. The cards are stacked against them. Excellent health care often cannot overcome the adverse effects of those determinants.

Evolution of Risk Assumption

Who assumes risk for health spending? In the past it has been hospitals, insurance companies, and patients. The physicians who decide whether to admit a patient to the hospital and who order tests and medications were assigned no risk for their decisions and orders. When physicians were subject to capitation, it typically did not result in significant cost reductions. Pay-for-performance programs paid for compliance with quality measures but were not focused on lowering costs. Now under the ACO program, after six years of assuming no risk, most ACOs will have to assume downside risk at some point in their new five-year CMS contracts, starting in 2019 and 2020. Assuming downside risk means that any losses below a specified minimum loss rate will have to be shared between Medicare and the provider. In post-2019 ACO programs, physician providers must assume their share of the losses. While this is CMS's goal, time will tell if the new approach reduces costs and improves quality more than occurred in the first six years of the ACO program.

Summary

Advances in medicine, monitoring for health care quality, evolving payment mechanisms, and forcing assumption of risk have brought us to today. Now care for a large percentage of the population will be based on the principles of the ACO. Our book will help guide you through this maelstrom, including how an ACO is set up, how it functions, and what are the keys to success. The relationship of the bundled payment programs and MIPS to ACOs is considered in detail. To orient you quickly, at the beginning of each chapter, I have written a brief description of content covered.

ACKNOWLEDGMENTS

To establish a successful accountable care organization takes a group of dedicated physicians and nurses. The same dedication is true for the authors writing this book. Once the topic was determined, I wrote the preface and overview, but then I needed expert input for chapters on specific aspects of the ACO.

I knew who to contact for many of the topics and was fortunate to know Joe Damore, vice president of strategy, innovation, and population health at Premier Inc., who helped me recruit experts for the other topics. For many years, Premier has been a training ground for tomorrow's health care leaders. Premier's experience with improving the quality of health care in numerous American institutions is legendary. My thanks to Joe for identifying Premier authors to write on these important areas.

Next, I would like to thank Chad Zimmerman, a health editor at Oxford University Press. His advice on the tone of the first chapter was helpful in making the writing more approachable. Chad also referred me to Johns Hopkins University Press because of its superb reputation as *the* health care policy publisher.

I want to convey my appreciation to Robin W. Coleman, acquisitions editor at Johns Hopkins University Press, who expressed interest and encouragement from the beginning of this endeavor. Through the lengthy review process and up to the final approval by their editorial boards, his patience and reassurance gave me the confidence to believe that we were on the right track. Robin also understood the importance of timely publication because CMS made significant changes to ACO policy in the last half of 2019.

And finally, I am grateful to my family who encouraged me to write this book and supported me with their continued interest. In particular, I want to express my appreciation to my journalist wife, Reggie, who edited my chapter and other parts of the book and continued to give me sound advice. Then to my children, Debby, Mike, and Dan, and their support team, Mark, Kate, and Karen, who asked, "Why don't you write a book on ACOs?" And so, I did.

Sadly, Dr. Peter A. Gross did not live to see the completion of the volume. He passed away in March 2020.

PATHWAYS TO A SUCCESSFUL
ACCOUNTABLE CARE ORGANIZATION

ONE

Essential Ingredients of a Successful Accountable Care Organization

PETER A. GROSS

The Hackensack Alliance is one of the most successful accountable care organizations (ACOs) in the United States, saving more than $193 million over six years. We are transparent with our numbers here in order to show how we performed financially and how compliant we were with the numerous quality measures. The keys to our success and the success of other ACOs are emphasized, and the evidence for these comments is carefully documented by references from the medical literature. The effects of the 2018 final rule changes from the Centers for Medicare and Medicaid Services (CMS) are also discussed.

Introduction: Health Care in the United States

How many times have you heard, "America has the best health care system in the world"? I wasn't sure who said that, so I went online to find someone quoted for the saying. The response was, "No documents match the query" (1). What then is the true story? Let's look at the facts.

Compare the United States with the developed nations in Europe, the Asia-Pacific, and North and South America who are members of the Organisation for Economic Co-operation and Development (OECD) (2). The United States has

- the most expensive per capita annual costs in a 2011 OECD report at $8,508, compared to the lowest cost of $3,182;
- the highest total expenditures of 17.7% on health care as a percentage of gross domestic product versus the lowest of 8.9% as reported in the *Los Angeles Times* in 2014 (3);
- the smallest percentage of population covered; and
- the lowest life expectancy at birth of less than 79 years versus an average of 82 years for all OECD countries.

The US is ranked 169th out of 224 countries for infant mortality in a government survey. When comparing older people to their counterparts abroad, a Commonwealth Fund survey of 11 countries showed that those in the US are sicker; are more likely to have trouble paying their medical bills; have more trouble getting necessary, timely care; and are more likely to use the emergency room for issues that primary care doctors can manage.

Finally, in the United States, a National Institutes of Health study found that approximately 200,000 Americans die each year from preventable medical errors, including facility-acquired conditions. And adverse drug events in the inpatient setting occur in approximately two million people annually and are responsible for increasing the length of stay by 1.7 to 4.6 days.

The US health care system has significant problems in access, cost, and quality. What can we do about it? It's not that we haven't tried. We started with diagnosis-related groups, where the goal was to decrease costs by decreasing the length of hospital stay. Following that, in the 1980s, health maintenance organizations were implemented to decrease costs by another approach, but no effort was made to increase the quality of care. Eventually, we switched to a greater focus on quality when Medicare and other payers instituted the pay-for-performance programs that encouraged compliance with a set of quality measures for heart attack, heart failure, community-acquired pneumonia, and surgical site infections. But the pay-for-performance programs didn't result in reducing costs. Consequently, should we focus on quality or costs? Ideally, we should develop a system that focuses on both.

Origin of the Concept of Accountable Care Organizations

In 2006, while attending a meeting of the Medicare Payment Advisory Commission, Dr. Elliott Fisher, from Dartmouth College, and others suggested that physicians should be accountable to their patients for both the cost and the quality of care (4). In addition, physicians should be incentivized to provide value-based care that would increase the quality of care while decreasing the cost. The financial incentives should partially replace the current fee-for-service method of payment. Organizations that would provide this accountable care would be known as accountable care organizations, or ACOs. Initial ACOs were started by the commercial payers. Then in 2011, Medicare, through CMS, entered the market and called for a Pioneer Savings Program for large health care institutions that had 15,000 or more patients. In 2012, CMS extended the concept by offering to contract with institutions that had 5,000 or more patients. It became known as the Medicare Shared Savings Program (MSSP) for CMS beneficiaries. CMS uses the term "beneficiaries" instead of "patients." We will use both interchangeably. The Pioneer ACOs were appointed in January 2012, while the first MSSP ACOs were designated in April 2012.

CMS's leadership role in promoting the accountable care organization concept has resulted in the formation of over 561 Medicare ACOs covering 10.5 million lives (5, 6). The leadership of the Medicare ACOs includes 171 physician group–led ACOs, 324 physician- and hospital-led ACOs, and 66 federally qualified health centers/rural health clinics (4, 6). There are also commercial ACOs. They actually predate Medicare ACOs. Commercial ACOs are clinically integrated networks of health care providers that are paid by commercial payers such as Blue Shield Blue Cross or by self-insured employers. The term *providers* includes physicians, nurse practitioners, physician assistants, and clinical nurse specialists. When commercial ACOs are added to the Medicare ACO numbers, we have more than 1,300 ACOs nationwide.

I should point out that in November and December 2018, CMS made significant changes to the organizational and financial structure as well as the management of ACOs. CMS's main intent was to have all ACOs assume downside risk on the cost of care. These changes are discussed throughout this chapter and other chapters in this book. In particular, CMS's major changes are described in the chapters on two-sided risk models by Brent Hardaway, Elyse Pegler, and Bryan Smith; quality measures by Guy D'Andrea and Kris Corwin; and coding by Glen Champlin and John Pitsikoulis.

ACO Types

CMS ACOs can assume one of several forms (3):

○ Independent physician group ACOs, which provide direct outpatient care
○ Physician group alliance ACOs, which include multiple physician groups that directly provide outpatient care
○ Expanded physician group ACOs, which directly provide outpatient care and have contracts for inpatient care
○ Independent hospital ACOs, which are single organizations that provide inpatient care
○ Hospital alliance ACOs, which include multiple organizations with at least one that directly provides inpatient care
○ Full-spectrum integrated ACOs, which include one or more organizations that directly provide all services
○ Certain critical access hospitals
○ Rural health clinics
○ Federally qualified health centers

ACO Application Process

Many Pioneer ACOs have dropped out of the program. Many lost monies and objected to using national cost trends rather than considering local cost trends. Some have converted to MSSPs, particularly Track 1. Therefore, we will focus on MSSPs. To apply to become a Medicare Shared Savings Program ACO, you need to check the CMS website (7) for the original requirements for Tracks 1, 1+, 2, and 3 (see also table 1.1 for a comparison of each track) and the new requirements for the new Basic and Enhanced Tracks (8–10). The final rule for the new tracks was issued December 21, 2018. A few policy changes were also issued in a November 1, 2018, release from CMS. Its determinants are described below and throughout the other chapters in this book. Be aware that all these changes are described under CMS's "Pathways to Success" web page.

Table 1.1. Comparison of the Medicare Shared Savings Program performance-based risk models by track

Issue	Track 1	Track 1+	Track 2	Track 3
Risk	One-sided	Two-sided	Two-sided	Two-sided
Agreement period	Two 3-year terms	Continuous	Continuous	Continuous
Assignment for reports	Prospective	Prospective	Prospective	Prospective
Assignment for financial reconciliation	Retrospective	Prospective	Retrospective	Prospective
Final sharing rate	Up to 50% based on quality score	Same as Track 1	Up to 60% based on quality score	Up to 75% based on quality score
Minimum savings rate (MSR)	2.0% to 3.9% depending on number of beneficiaries	Same as Track 2	Choice of symmetrical MSR/MLR in 0.5% increments between 0.5% and 2.0%	Same as Track 2
Minimum loss rate (MLR)	Not applicable	See MSR options	See MSR options	See MSR options
Performance payment limit	10%	Same as Track 1	15%	20%
Shared savings	First dollar sharing once MSR is met or exceeded	Same as Track 1	Same as Track 1	Same as Track 1
Shared loss rate	Not applicable	Fixed at 30%. Applied to first dollar loss once MLR is met or exceeded.	Similar to Track 1+ but range is 40%–60%	Similar to Track 1+ but range is 40%–75%
Loss sharing limit	Not applicable	Limit on amount depends on options or 8% of fee-for-service revenue.	Limit varies between 5% and 10% depending on year. Losses below annual limit are not shared.	Limit of 15% of historical benchmark. Losses below limit are not shared.
Skilled nursing facility 3-day rule waiver	Not applicable	ACO may elect to apply	Not applicable	ACO may elect to apply

Note: Benchmarking is rebased or reset at beginning of each agreement period with phase-in of a regional adjustment for all tracks. For additional information on shared loss rate, loss sharing limit, and repayment mechanisms (type and amount), refer to the Centers for Medicare and Medicaid Services fact sheet *New Accountable Care Organization Model Opportunity: Medicare ACO Track 1+ Model*, https://www.cms.gov/Medicare/Medicare-Fee-for-Service-Payment/sharedsavingsprogram/Downloads/New-Accountable-Care-Organization-Model-Opportunity-Fact-Sheet.pdf (updated July 2017; accessed November 14, 2019).

Supporting documents needed are noted on the CMS website. CMS will provide guidance and templates. For old Tracks 1+, 2, and 3 and the new Basic and Enhanced Tracks, physicians are subject to downside risk, which means they are required to share in losses incurred beyond the minimum loss rate. CMS recommends that you indicate your repayment mechanism should you incur losses. Also note, the old Track 1 and the new Basic Track Levels A and B are the only tracks with no downside risk. CMS wants all ACOs eventually to assume downside risk.

You will need to decide whether you want to apply for one of the five Basic Tracks or the one Enhanced Track. Those ACO sites already in the old Track 1+, 2, and 3 will finish out their contracts with CMS. If you want to continue in the MSSP, you would then apply for one of the five Basic Tracks or the Enhanced Track:

A. Basic Track Levels A and B
- One-sided models: ACOs can be part of Levels A and B for one to three years depending on certain restrictions. Not an option for most existing ACOs.
- Potential gains: First dollar savings at a rate of 40% based on quality performance. Gain not to exceed 10% of updated benchmark.

B. Basic Track Level C
- Potential gains: Once minimum savings rate is met or exceeded, first dollar savings will be at a rate of up to 50% based on quality performance. Savings not to exceed 10% of updated benchmark.
- Potential losses: Shared losses once minimum loss rate is met or exceeded, and first dollar losses at a rate of 30%. Loss not to exceed 2% of ACO participant revenue capped at 1% of updated benchmark.

C. Basic Track Level D
- Potential gains: Same as Level C.
- Potential losses: First dollar losses at 30%. Loss not to exceed 4% and capped at 2% of updated benchmark.

D. Basic Track Level E
- Potential gains: Same as Level C.
- Potential losses: First dollar losses at 30%. Loss not to exceed 8% and capped at 4% of updated benchmark.

E. Enhanced Track (similar to Track 3)
- Potential gains: Once minimum savings rate is met or exceeded, first dollar savings will be up to 75% based on quality performance. Gain not to exceed 20% of updated benchmark.
- Potential losses: Shared losses once minimum loss is rate met or exceeded, first dollar losses will be at a rate of 1 minus the final sharing rate with minimum shared loss rate of 40% and maximum of 75%. Loss not to exceed 15% of updated benchmark.

Annually, you may elect to enter a higher risk level except for those in Basic Track Level E and those in the Enhanced Track. Applicants for the new Basic and Enhanced Tracks had a start date of July 1, 2019. Previous applicants whose second three-year contract expired December 31, 2018, had their contract extended six months to July 1, 2019.

While the new Basic Tracks and Enhanced Track are what is currently required, I will keep referring to the old Tracks 1, 1+, 2, and 3 because they are the ones that all ACOs have used and have had experience with for the past six years (2012–2018). As the new Basic and Enhanced Tracks have not been used yet, there is no experience with them that can be cited. Organizations in the old Track 1+ and Track 3; the new Basic Track Levels C, D, and E; and the Enhanced Track (modeled after the old Track 3) may apply for the skilled nursing facility (SNF) three-day rule waiver. They require SNF Affiliate Agreements and an Agreement Crosswalk. CMS guidance is also available for these agreements. Under the new Pathways to Success, the Bipartisan Budget Act provided those in Basic Levels C, D, and E and the Enhanced Track with a broader three-day SNF waiver, expanded telehealth services, and beneficiary incentive programs that provide financial incentives for beneficiaries to facilitate their medical and preventive care.

In addition to the old four tracks, the Next Generation ACO model was popular (11, 12). The model was best suited for groups who are experienced with managing care for populations. The agreement period was for three years with options to renew for two one-year periods. A choice is to be made between Risk Arrangement A or B. For Arrangement A, shared savings and losses are up to 80% and for Arrangement B, shared savings and losses are up to 100%. The historical benchmark is a one-year calculation, instead of three, with a discount and a one-year regional trend. It is reset at the beginning of each year. Different payment mechanisms are available for losses, such as fee-for-service, capitation, and per-beneficiary-per-month. Indirect medical education and disproportionate share hospital payments are included. Next Generation ACOs can use three waivers that relate to expanding telehealth usage, more flexibility with post-hospital discharge home visits, and avoidance of the three-day skilled nursing facility rule. Financial benchmarks are set prospectively at the beginning of a performance year.

To initiate an application, a track should be selected and a governing board created to execute the functions of the ACO. One board member must be a Medicare beneficiary. Other members' job responsibilities should be carefully described. Then operating committees should be appointed.

The provider participants must supply taxpayer identification numbers (TINs) and sign participation agreements. The agreements are modeled after the MSSP recommendations. The agreement for electronic funds transfer authorization should include, for example, the organization's identifying information, legal business name, TIN, financial institution information, and authorized or delegated official.

For those ACOs renewing contracts after three years, a renewal application process is available on the CMS website. New contracts signed after 2018 extend to five years.

Track 1, which has no downside risk, is no longer available for new ACOs starting in 2019–2020. A somewhat similar track is now available under the Basic Track, Levels A and B, for only one to three years.

In general, the steps surrounding the application process look like this:

1. Complete a Notice of Intent to Apply.
2. Obtain a CMS User ID.
3. Submit the application using the application toolkit and the process discussed earlier.
4. Respond to requests for information regarding the application.
5. Sign the MSSP ACO participation agreement and the data use agreement.

The CMS timelines for due dates of these steps should be checked for the year you are applying as they may change from the previous year.

ACO Evaluation Process

After receiving an acceptance from CMS, how will the ACO be evaluated by you, CMS, or commercial enterprises? There are both financial considerations that emphasize resource use and quality considerations that examine compliance with a significant number of quality measures. Transparency of results is one of the goals of CMS in the MSSP. For example, tables 1.2 and 1.3 report the way the Hackensack Alliance ACO performed for costs by practice group and for quality measures, respectively, for the entire ACO (13, 14).

As with most initial MSSP ACOs, we opted for being in Track 1, which meant if we reduced resource use, we would potentially be able to share with CMS in the savings. However, if we spent more than CMS projected for us and had losses, we were not responsible for paying CMS part of the losses. If the ACO had savings, the amount of savings that is divided with CMS would depend on the quality score. This is one of the primary differences between MSSP ACOs and the managed care plans of the 1990s that solely focused on resource-use reduction. The quality of care provided was not a consideration in the 1990s. The current approach is part of the Triple Aim goal promoted by Donald Berwick (15). The Triple Aim promotes better care for the individual, better health for the population, and reduced growth of expenses. Another connecting concept often used is Value = Quality/Cost.

Financial Considerations

Each quarter, CMS sends the ACOs the claim and claim line feeds (CCLFs). They detail the claims submitted by providers, namely, physicians, nurse practitioners, physician assistants, hospitals, skilled nursing facilities, and other service providers. The CCLFs are sent to a data analytics firm who arrange the data into a form that can be used. The analysis is sent to a health care management consultant (in our case, it was Premier Inc., Health Endeavors, and Verisk), who review the data and point out areas that need attention. The data analysis describes the results for the ACO as a whole (table 1.2) and is about the practice groups identified by their TIN or about individual providers by national provider identifier (not shown) within a TIN. The data analyzed for the quality measure performance of the entire ACO is extremely useful (table 1.3). Through Premier Inc. we are regularly compared to a group of approximately 30 other ACOs and to all MSSP ACOs in the country. A somewhat similar analysis is performed by the National Association for ACOs. Both show potential areas for improvement. The key clinical findings are presented to our providers.

It should be noted that the CCLFs may not include some patients (i.e., beneficiaries). These are the patients who initially opted out of having their data shared with the ACO. For the Hackensack Alliance ACO, that concern was a small number, approximately 2% of the total number of assigned patients. Under the new Pathways to Success, the opt-in rules have been changed. Also under Pathways, a beneficiary already aligned with a physician can join the physician's ACO by being assigned prospectively.

In some instances, we were able to analyze our CCLFs by practice group (i.e., TIN) as shown in table 1.2. The three largest groups, identified by practice codes A, B, and C, had reduced hospital admissions, reduced readmissions, and reduced emergency room visits compared to the ACO norm for that resource use. Not all TINs performed as well, but most TINs did perform better than the ACO norm. It is important to point out that office visits were considerably above the ACO norm. This excess is good because it meant that physicians saw their patients

Table 1.2. Admissions and visits per 1,000 plus cost and utilization summary for all practices and individual practices

Practice code	Number of beneficiaries[a]	Relative risk score[b]	Inpatient admissions	ACO norm	Readmissions rate[c]	ACO readmissions rate norm	Office visits	ACO office visits norm	ER visits	ACO ER visits norm	Average cost per member ($)	Medicare per-member per-month cost ($)	Medicare per-member per-month cost ($) norm
All	13,385	1.07	216	317	0.12	0.16	12,716	9,632	503	835	21,540	879	858
A	1,538	0.94	137	317	0.12	0.16	12,954	9,632	320	835	17,284	720	858
B	1,176	0.90	153	317	0.06	0.16	11,992	9,632	381	835	15,905	663	858
C	2,219	0.86	149	317	0.10	0.16	11,894	9,632	378	835	15,838	660	858
D	628	0.91	165	317	0.11	0.16	10,995	9,632	333	835	16,720	696	858
E	257	0.91	158	317	0.09	0.16	12,383	9,632	331	835	18,497	771	858
F	436	1.94	471	317	0.13	0.16	12,954	9,632	1,063	835	44,923	1,872	858
G	36	1.43	319	317	0.00	0.16	17,250	9,632	736	835	35,542	1,473	858
H	877	1.10	219	317	0.11	0.16	11,478	9,632	471	835	22,238	926	858
I	4,505	1.20	274	317	0.14	0.16	13,552	9,632	647	835	25,779	1,074	858
J	33	1.95	803	317	0.28	0.16	13,348	9,632	1,500	835	48,465	2,019	858
K	21	1.48	405	317	0.31	0.16	5,119	9,632	571	835	31,220	1,301	858
L	381	0.88	136	317	0.13	0.16	13,333	9,632	365	835	16,043	668	858
M	604	0.96	176	317	0.11	0.16	13,430	9,632	382	835	18,287	762	858
N	77	1.20	292	317	0.08	0.16	14,649	9,632	500	835	25,810	1,075	858
O	76	0.76	169	317	0.05	0.16	10,331	9,632	599	835	15,867	661	858
P	39	0.77	115	317	0.00	0.16	11,371	9,632	551	835	12,965	540	858
Q	176	1.18	315	317	0.10	0.16	15,923	9,632	514	835	23,432	976	858
R	148	0.86	128	317	0.19	0.16	11,111	9,632	324	835	14,349	600	858
S	17	0.99	206	317	0.00	0.16	10,029	9,632	471	835	32,939	1,372	858

Source: Data from Verisk Analytics for the period of July 2012 to June 2014.
[a]Total number of beneficiaries should be at least 50, but preferably 100 or more, before drawing conclusions about making efforts to improve.
[b]Total risk within a population using Model 125.
[c]Readmissions are reported as an inpatient readmission rate, not per 1,000.

more often than the ACO norm in order to manage chronic problems and avoid hospitalization or emergency room admission. Finally, the per-member-per-month costs were less than the ACO norm for most, but not all groups. The biggest ACO expenses usually come from unnecessary hospital admissions, readmissions, and emergency room visits. That, then, was a reasonable place to look when assessing resource use. In Hackensack's case, these reductions happened from the inception of our ACO without any encouragement or instructions to the providers. The reductions probably occurred because the physicians enrolled were already efficient through their offices by being recognized as a patient-centered medical home (PCMH) by the National Committee for Quality Assurance (NCQA). Not only can a practice be recognized as a PCMH, but an entire ACO can be accredited as such by NCQA. Dr. Joshua Bennett describes PCMHs in detail in chapter 2.

Practice groups and individual providers received information on their performance by newsletter and at ACO meetings. Physicians are very competitive. If they realize that another group performs better, then showing them their results is one of the most efficient methods for fostering change and improvement.

Quality Considerations

Next, Hackensack showed its providers the quality measures by which they would be judged (table 1.3). The measures were approved by the National Quality Forum (NQF), and most of them are evidence-based, particularly the measures in the last two domains. Chapter 4 on quality measures by Guy D'Andrea and Kris Corwin addresses how the NQF establishes the measures and determines their reliability and effectiveness. CMS has assigned 33 measures to be assessed by each ACO in the MSSP. The 33 measures are divided into four domains:

- Patient/caregiver experience: 6 measures
- Care coordination/patient safety: 5 measures
- Preventive health: 8 measures
- At-risk population (with five subdomains and 14 measures total):

a. Diabetes: 6 individual measures and 1 group measure

b. Hypertension: 1 measure

c. Ischemic vascular disease: 2 measures

d. Heart failure: 1 measure

e. Coronary heart disease: 2 individual measures and 1 group measure

Table 1.3 is an example of how Hackensack's ACO scored on quality measures. It shows the number of points awarded for each measure or composite measure out of the possible maximum number of points that can be assigned to successful implementation of the measure. The table also shows the 90th percentile target as well as the median rate for all ACOs. For some measures, such as measure 27, the goal is to have a low value rather than a high one. Hence, for diabetic patients, a hemoglobin A1c above 9% is considered poor control. For your population, you would want to aim for the finding of poor control at 10% or less.

In each ACO, CMS will survey some patients for the 12 measures in the first two domains, namely, patient/caregiver experience and care coordination/patient safety. ACOs are responsible for reporting the 22 measures in the last two domains, namely, preventive health and at-risk populations. These measures correspond to the old measures of the group practice reporting option. (See chapter 5 on quality data collection by Kris Gates and chapter 6 on quality audits by Mitchel Easton.)

Besides the obvious patient benefit of having all these measures successfully implemented, perfect implementation of the measures entitles the ACO to receive 50% of the savings achieved for the year. When implementation falls short of 100%, the percent compliance is multiplied by 50% to determine the percentage the ACO will receive. For example, if quality measure compliance is 89%, the percentage of the savings that the ACO can claim is 89% × 50%, or 44.5%, rather than 50%. The remaining 50% accrues to CMS.

Subsequent quality measure sets have been significantly reduced in the number of measures, particularly the 2019–2020 set (see chapter 4). The reduction was designed to reduce the administrative burden. Of

Table 1.3. 2014 quality measure results for the Hackensack Alliance ACO

ACO measure number	Description of measures	Hackensack ACO performance rate (%)	Points earned/total possible points	Median rate (%) of all ACOs[a]	90th percentile benchmark
	Domain: patient/caregiver experience				
1	Getting timely care, appointments, and information	77	1.70/2	81	90
2	How well your doctors communicate	92	2.00/2	93	90
3	Patients' rating of doctor	91	2.00/2	92	90
4	Access to specialist	87	1.85/2	84	90
5	Health promotion and education	60	1.85/2	58	61
6	Shared decision making	71	0.00/2	75	77
7	Health status/functional status	69	2.00/2	71	NA
	Points earned in domain		11.40/14		
	Domain: care coordination/patient safety				
8	Risk standardized, all condition readmission[b]	16[c]	2.00/2	15	15
9	Ambulatory surgery center admission: COPD or asthma in older adults	1.03[c,d]	1.40/2	1.03	0.27
10	Ambulatory surgery center admission: heart failure	1.19[c,d]	1.10/2	1.18	0.38
11	Percentage of primary care providers who qualified for electronic health record incentive[e]	78	3.40/4	80	91
12	Medication reconciliation	94	2.00/2	92	90
13	Falls: screening for fall risk	70	1.85/2	45	73
	Points earned in domain		11.75/14		
	Domain: preventive health				
14	Influenza immunization	80	1.70/2	58	100
15	Pneumococcal immunization	73	1.55/2	57	100
16	Adult weight screening and follow-up	92	1.70/2	68	100
17	Tobacco use assessment and cessation information	98	2.00/2	91	90
18	Depression screening	67	2.00/2	37	52
19	Colorectal cancer screening	74	2.00/2	58	100
20	Mammography screening	76	2.00/2	63	100
21	Proportion of adults who had blood pressure screened in past two years	95	2.00/2	59	90
	Points earned in domain		14.95/16		

	Domain: at-risk population				
	Subdomain: diabetes				
	Beneficiaries with diabetes who met all of the following criteria:	39	2.00/2[f]	26	37
22	Hemoglobin A1c control (HbA1c) (<8%)	79	—	26	NA
23	Low density lipoprotein (LDL) (<100 mg/dL)	68	—	26	NA
24	Blood pressure (BP) <140/90	76	—	26	NA
25	Tobacco non-use	92	—	26	NA
26	Aspirin use	98	—	26	NA
27	Percentage of beneficiaries with diabetes whose HbA1c is in poor control (>9%)	9.60	2.00/2	18	10
	Subdomain: hypertension				
28	Percentage of beneficiaries with hypertension whose BP is <140/90	82	2.00/2	69	80
	Subdomain: ischemic vascular disease (IVD)				
29	Percentage of beneficiaries with IVD with complete lipid profile and LDL control is <100mg/dL	67	2.00/2	59	79
30	Percentage of beneficiaries who use aspirin or other antithrombotic	93	1.85/2	85	98
	Subdomain: heart failure				
31	Beta-blocker therapy for left ventricular systolic dysfunction (LVSD)	97	2.00/2	88	90
	Subdomain: coronary artery disease (CAD)				
	Percentage of beneficiaries with CAD who met all of the following criteria:	78	2.00/2[g]	69	80
32	Drug therapy for lowering LDL cholesterol	80	—	69	NA
33	Angiotensin-converting enzyme inhibitor or angiotensin II receptor blocker therapy for patients with CAD and diabetes and/or LVSD	89	—	69	NA
	Points earned in domain		13.85/14		

[a] The total number of ACOs studied ranged from 322 to 333, depending on the measure assessed.
[b] A single summary risk standardized readmission rate for measure 8 is derived from the volume-weighted results of five different specialty models.
[c] For measures 8, 9, 10, and 27, a lower performance rate indicates better performance.
[d] Measures 9 and 10 show a ratio of observed over expected rate. Hence, a ratio >1.00 indicates a higher than expected admission rate and poorer quality.
[e] Measure 11 is double-weighted because of the importance of the electronic health record incentive program.
[f] Composite score for diabetes subdomain includes measures 22–26.
[g] Composite score for coronary artery disease subdomain includes measures 32 and 33.

note is that those ACOs who bear risk (i.e., Basic Levels C, D, and E and Enhanced Track) will qualify as an advanced alternative payment model (Advanced APM) and be exempt from many of the Quality Payment Program requirements. Those in Basic Levels A and B do not qualify as an Advanced APM.

Savings Calculation

The actual savings achieved by an ACO is determined by a complex calculation shown in table 1.4. The numbers shown are for the second year (i.e., 2014) of Hackensack Alliance ACO's CMS contract. Going back to the beginning of our ACO, we saved $10,747,668 in 2012–2013. It should be noted that our first year was 21 months long from April 2012 through December 2013. The amount CMS shared with our ACO was $5,266,357. It was close to 50% because our quality score was 100%. The first year was considered a reporting year for the quality score; it was not a performance or compliance year. We received credit for reporting that we were monitoring the measures, not that we complied with them.

The second year was a calendar year from January through December 2014 (table 1.4). The assigned beneficiaries line shows the number of patients followed by the ACO at the end of the year. Determining the beneficiary population at that time is called "retrospective assign-

Table 1.4. Shared savings calculations for performance year 2 (2014)

a.	Assigned beneficiaries	15,603
b.	Person-years	15,158
c.	Per capita expenditures benchmark ($)	13,099
d.	Per capita expenditures actual ($)	12,672
e.	Total benchmark expenditures ($) (b×c)	198,546,103
f.	Total actual expenditures ($)	192,081,207
g.	Total savings ($) (e−f)	6,464,895
h.	Minimum saving rate (%)	2.70
i.	Minimum savings rate ($) (h×e)	5,312,846
j.	Potential net savings ($) (g/2)	3,232,448
k.	Quality performance sharing rate (%) (out of a possible 50%)	50
l.	Hackensack's final quality score (%)	89.4
m.	Hackensack's final sharing rate (%) (k×l)	44.7
n.	Interim savings ($) (g×m)	2,890,804
o.	Less sequester adjustment ($)	57,816
p.	Final net earned savings performance payment ($) (n−o)	2,832,988

ment." "Prospective assignment" would indicate the number of patients followed at the beginning of the year. Another factor is that CMS prefers using person-years because it more accurately accounts for the number of months that a patient is in the ACO.

It should be noted that a beneficiary is assigned to a primary care physicians when they have at least one primary care visit from an ACO physician. The primary care physician is defined as someone who specializes in internal medicine, general practice, family practice, or geriatric medicine. The determination is based on a two-step process. First, the beneficiary has to receive the plurality of their primary care visits from the physician. The second step occurs when the provider is not a primary care physician. Then assignment can be made to the ACO if the provider is a physician specialist, nurse practitioner, clinical nurse specialist, or physician assistant. Under Pathways to Success, additional positions are considered eligible clinicians. They are physical therapists, occupational therapists, qualified speech-language pathologists, qualified audiologists, clinical psychologist, and registered dieticians or nutrition professionals. Pathways also permits an ACO to annually select prospective or retrospective assignment of beneficiaries.

The next value on table 1.4 is the per capita historical benchmark, set by CMS at $13,099 for the Hackensack Alliance ACO. The historical benchmark reflects the average expenses for the prior three years. The three years are weighted differently. For example, the 2009 historical expenditures are weighted 10%; 2010, 30%; and 2011, 60%. The federal Office of the Actuary also adjusts the composite benchmark annually in order to reflect changes in beneficiary characteristics and the amount of growth in per capita expenditures. Hackensack's total historical expenditure benchmark was $198,546,103. Under the new Pathways, the historical benchmark will be composed of both national and regional financial data. Depending on how you compare to peers in your geographic region will determine whether the addition of regional expenditures is a benefit or detriment to your historical benchmark calculation.

The actual per capita expenses were less at $12,672. The actual per capita expenses are multiplied by the person-years to determine the total actual expenditures, which are $192,081,207. If you do the multiplication yourself the numbers come out close but not identical. The slight difference may be related to the number of cents in the per capita numbers that are not shown. Nevertheless, the difference between the total historical benchmark and the total actual expenses is $6,464,895.

The next hurdle to overcome is the minimum savings rate (MSR) (16). CMS estimated that there is random variation in the numbers due to chance. They estimated that random variation was approximately 2%–4%, depending on the number of beneficiaries in the program. The larger the number of beneficiaries, the smaller the MSR percentage. The minimum savings rate accounts for the variation on the upside and a minimum loss rate accounts for variation on the downside. Considering the Hackensack program, the MSR was 2.7%. The MSR multiplied by the total historical benchmark (2.7% × $198,546,103) equaled an MSR hurdle of $5,312,846. In order to participate in the savings, any ACO has to exceed the MSR. Having savings of $6,464,895 was the first step.

The second step is to calculate 50% of the savings, which is $3,232,448. That totals the potential savings CMS will send to Hackensack for being cost efficient. However, the payment depends on the quality score. That final quality score in 2014 was 89.4%. To calculate the percentage eligible for determining our shared savings, the two are multiplied (i.e., 50% × 89.4%) which is 44.7%. Therefore, Hackensack qualified for 44.7% of the total savings of $6,464,895, or $2,890,804.

The last item to be deducted from the savings is the sequester. That amount in 2014 is from when the federal government was shut down. The sequester came to $57,816, which is deducted from the above savings to yield $2,832,988—the amount that CMS paid to the Hackensack Alliance ACO for the 2014 effort.

As a side note, other factors affect both the total historical and actual expenditures. Those numbers depend on the distribution of assigned patients in your ACO. CMS uses four enrollment categories for its beneficiaries:

○ End-stage renal disease, which are the most expensive and usually the smallest number of beneficiaries in your ACO

- Disabled
- Aged and dual eligible for Medicare and Medicaid
- Aged and non–dual eligible, having Medicare only

The aged, non-dual group usually composes the highest percentage of patients, in Hackensack's case 86.5% of all beneficiaries. They are the least expensive per patient, but this category generates the largest percentage of expenditures because it has the largest percentage of patients. Keep this in mind as you decide where to place your initial priorities for reducing utilization or resource use. Of note is that indirect medical education, disproportionate share hospital, and uncompensated care payments are not included in the ACO expenditure numbers.

Risk Scoring

It is also important to consider your risk score because it affects the value of the historical benchmark. CMS uses a hierarchical condition category (HCC) to risk score your beneficiaries and it's done retrospectively. Each year, CMS updates the HCC for changes in health status and demographic factors that appear in the originally assigned beneficiaries. The risk scores can go up or down and depend on the diagnostic codes that the providers bill CMS for their services. Risk scoring is covered in greater depth by Glen Champlin in chapter 10. Under Pathways, there is an allowance for risk score growth over the contract period.

Distribution of Net Savings to the ACO Providers

If you have a savings above the MSR, then you need to determine how it will be distributed to the participants in the ACO. A few factors have to be considered. The easiest is to distribute the savings based on the percentage of CMS beneficiaries in the practice's taxpayer identification number or assigned to the individual national provider identifier. Other considerations are the quality score of the TIN or provider; utilization or resources used by the TIN or provider; good citizenship, such as cooperation and helpfulness; and educational credits acquired. You will also need to repay your debts for operating the ACO, and you might want to put some savings aside for future operating expenses in case the next year's savings are less.

ACOs Record of Cost Savings to Date

In Year 1 of the MSSP, 53 of 220 ACOs (24.2%) achieved sufficient savings to exceed the MSR and earn shared savings. In Year 2, 98 of 355 ACOs (27.5%) earned shared savings. In each of these years, approximately another quarter of the ACOs had cost savings but did not exceed their MSRs; consequently, no savings were earned. Over subsequent years, the percentage with earned savings has gradually increased. For the first two years, only 38 of 353 (10.8%) were able to generate savings two years in a row (according to a memo from Holly Wittenberg, Avalere Health, February 2016). The Hackensack Alliance ACO was part of that group.

Our ACO has generated savings six years in a row (table 1.5). It is interesting to point out that over those six years, our actual per capita expenditures have stayed relatively stable, while the historical benchmark per capita expenditures, for the most part, have increased. As a result, our cost savings have increased each year to a total savings in the fourth year of $50.5 million, the third highest in the country. The fifth year was different as the information used by CMS changed. As a result, our benchmark and actual expenditures both decreased. The total savings over six years was $194,070,274.

What Worked for Us

1. *Selecting the right physicians*: We picked physicians whose practices were recognized by NCQA as a patient-centered medical home (see chapter 2 by Dr. Joshua Bennett). The thinking was that they were already accustomed to focusing on complying with quality measures and were efficient utilizers of resources. We said we would accept anyone else into our ACO as long as they became recognized as a PCMH by NCQA

Table 1.5. Hackensack Alliance ACO: Comparison of key results over six years

	Factor Compared	2012+2013[a]	2014	2015	2016	2017	2018
a.	Assigned beneficiaries	13,911	15,603	23,156	29,546	35,513	38,660
b.	Person-years	13,528	15,158	22,522	28,809	34,724	37,839
c.	Per capita expenditures benchmark ($)	12,547	13,099	13,507	13,917	12,866	12,868
d.	Per capita expenditures actual ($)	12,302	12,672	12,026	12,163	11,609	11,564
e.	Decrease in per capita expenditures ($) (c−d)	245	427	1,481	1,753	1,257	1,304
f.	Total benchmark expenditures ($)	279,469,265	198,546,103	304,196,419	400,924,471	446,762,619	486,907,951
g.	Total actual expenditures ($)	268,721,597	192,081,207	270,843,109	350,413,008	403,115,528	437,562,125
h.	Total savings in expenditures ($) (f−g)	10,747,668	6,464,896	33,353,310	50,511,463	43,647,091	49,345,826
i.	Initial sharing rate (%)	50	50	50	50	50	50
j.	Quality score (%)	100	89.43	95.70	91.92	84.90	89.37
k.	Final sharing rate (%) (i×j)	50	44.7	47.9	46.0	42.5	44.7
l.	Total savings in expenditures ($)	10,747,668	6,464,896	33,353,310	50,511,463	43,647,091	49,345,826
m.	Savings after quality adjustment ($) (k×l)	5,373,834	2,890,804	15,960,080	23,214,944	18,528,314	22,048,963
n.	Sequestration adjustment ($)	107,477	57,816	319,202	464,299	370,566	440,979
o.	Net earned performance payment from CMS ($) (m−n)	5,266,357	2,832,988	15,640,878	22,750,645	18,157,748	21,607,983

Note: Most remarkable is the decrease in per capita expenditures (line e) compared with the benchmark expenditures (line c). This progressive decrease went from $245 to $1,753 per capita over four years and is still significant in the fifth year and sixth years. Also note that the benchmark expenditures actually increased over time. Expenditures were higher in the first performance year because it was 21 months long rather than 12 months. Actual per capita expenditures were the lowest in the sixth year (2018). Beginning in 2017, benchmarks were lower because a regional factor was included, the percentage of aged non-dual beneficiaries increased, and the CMS calculation methodology changed.

[a]The first performance year of the CMS ACO contract represents April 2012 through December 2013. Lines a, b, c, d, and e in this column represent the data for 2013 only.

within one year. We would pay to have a consultant help them get certified. They also had to use an electronic medical record. If these two objectives were not met within a year, they could not remain in the ACO.

2. Next, we focused on *hiring nurse care coordinators*. The person in charge of recruitment is a nurse practitioner trained at Duke in care coordination. She was very selective in hiring nurse coordinators. They had to be personable, able to get along with difficult personalities, and experienced in nursing. They focused on the high-risk patients. Hiring nurse coordinators was the second most important key to our success. (See chapter 3 by the creator of our nurse coordinator program, Denise Patriaco.)

3. *Compliance with the 33 CMS quality measures* was critical to the health of the patients and to determine whether the ACO shared in the cost savings (see chapter 4 on quality measurement, chapter 9 on selecting a data analytic company, and chapter 15 on the value of ACO consultants).

4. *Availability of data analytics*, we knew, was important for assessing our performance. However, we had a false start with the initial data analytic company that we hired. We finally settled on using Premier Inc. to interpret our results, which were analyzed by Verisk, Healthfirst, and Milliman later. The CCLFs and financial reconciliation reports from CMS were sent to these companies for analysis. The assessment of compliance with the quality measures was a collaborative effort of our data manager, nurse coordinators, and Health Endeavors. (See chapter 9 on the selection process for data analytics.)

5. The *role of risk scores and regional differences in expenditures* influenced our historic benchmark expenditures and actual expenditures. Our risk scores were higher than average, and our local expenses were higher than other regions, which proved to be an advantage in determining the cost savings. (See chapter 10 on importance of coding for optimal risk scores.)

Ingredients of Success from the Literature

We have reviewed the literature and present what some other investigators thought influenced the success of ACOs.

Encourage Use of the Patient-Centered Medical Home Model

Several pundits seem to agree that the recognition of being a patient-centered medical home prepared a physician's practice to be more efficient in dealing with utilization of the health care system, such as reducing unnecessary hospital admission, readmissions, and emergency room visits. Secondly, the PCMH model promotes the use of additional personnel to coordinate the care of the patient. Finally, the PCMH model prepares the physician and the office to comply with a list of quality measures that improve communication with the patient and offer preventive services such as immunization and colonoscopy.

At least three organizations offer medical home recognition that recognizes a physician's practice as a PCMH. The three are the National Committee for Quality Assurance, The Joint Commission, and the Accreditation Association for Ambulatory Health Care. NCQA also offers a separate accreditation for ACOs as a medical home unit. NCQA is the program most often selected for PCMH recognition.

Be aware that the effectiveness of using the PCMH structure is somewhat controversial. The reasons may relate to different amounts of compliance with the PCMH requirements and recommendations. The issues are

- use of care coordination,
- use of preventive health services,
- identifying the high-risk patients,
- promoting efforts to reduce utilization,
- focusing on an approach to providing patient-centered care, and
- seeking one of the levels of recognition (1, 2, or 3).

Provide Care Coordination

Appreciate that different patients need different levels of care:

- Two to three percent of your beneficiaries are complex and require individual case management. They are 40% of your costs.

- Five to seven percent of your population are also complex but can be managed by primary care providers (17).
- Twenty to twenty-five percent of your population can be managed with disease management by virtual/telephonic approaches.
- One hundred percent of your population requires an annual visit for a wellness and prevention program.

Nurse coordinators play a key role in managing these four levels of care with the physicians. You should use the data from the quarterly CMS CCLF reports to identify areas of high cost and high utilization. Focus on improving the cited areas.

Create a High-Value Culture

If you already have a high-value culture, you are ahead of the game. A high-value culture is usually a result of the organization's leadership promoting a drive for high quality in patient care over time (18). It is reflected in more than the mission, vision, and value statements. It is evident in the attitudes of the senior leaders in their day-to-day statements and activities. Many high-value organizations have already managed risk or participated in pay-for-performance programs.

Promote Physician and Clinical Practice Engagement

The governance structure should be composed of leaders of physician practices and hospital representatives, when the hospital administration is part of the ACO. Other staff members should be included, too, such as the nurse care coordinators and physician office staff representatives. Depending on the ownership structure, post-acute care representatives from nursing homes, home care, and hospice should be added to the governance structure. Broad representation will facilitate coordination of implementation strategies. Pick the passionate providers to maintain momentum in the improvement process. Drive the bus by fueling it with acquired data that is fed back to all providers. (See chapter 13 by Dr. Morey Menacker on primary care and chapter 14 by Dr. Thomas Kloos on practice transformation.)

Monitor Post-Acute Care

This area includes use of skilled nursing facilities, long-term care facilities, home health, hospice, and hospital outpatient facilities. Providers and patients need to collaborate and determine the optimal location for each patient following hospitalization. (See chapter 8 by Andy Edeburn on post-acute care.)

Be aware of perverse incentives interfering with cost efficiency. For example, a hospital's incentive under diagnosis-related groups is to discharge the patient as soon as possible since they are paid a certain rate based on diagnosis. The nursing home is paid by CMS for a specific length of stay; consequently, their incentive is to keep the patient until the specified length of stay is reached.

Identify High-Risk Patients

Use a system that identifies the high-risk patients. Their numbers will be relatively small, but their expenses are relatively large. Create the list of high-risk patients from claims and clinical data. These are the 5% of patients that will need extensive care management.

Develop a Chronic Disease Management Program

The chronic diseases to focus on are diabetes mellitus, congestive heart failure, chronic obstructive pulmonary disease, and chronic kidney disease. Within each group practice, create disease registries and adopt pre-existing evidence-based algorithms for better chronic disease management. (See chapter 16 by Seth Edwards on the Comprehensive Primary Care Plus Initiative.)

Use Performance on Quality, Utilization, and Other Measures as Potential Criteria for Compensation

- Every 3, 6, or 12 months show providers their individual or group performance on these measures.
- Compare quality and utilization measure results with other ACOs at the national or state level.
- Assess accuracy of coding for risk.
- Assess compliance with behavioral norms.
- Acquire new ideas from peers and other national organizations.

Avoid Low-Value Care

It has been estimated that one-fifth of all health care is unnecessary—that is, patient care with no net benefit (19–21). The top five low-value health services noted by the Task Force on Low-Value Care are

- diagnostic testing and imaging for low-risk patients prior to low-risk surgery,
- population-based vitamin D screening,
- prostate-specific antigen screening in men ages 75 and older,
- imaging for acute low-back pain for the first six weeks after onset, unless clinical warning signs are present, and
- use of more expensive branded drugs instead of generic drugs with the same activity.

The task force describes a total of 44 low-value health services that cost over $500 million in 2014. These unnecessary services can increase the risk of cancer from radiation, result in incidental findings that lead the clinician on a wild-goose chase, and lead to complications such as bleeding or infection. You should review the recommendations and implement where appropriate.

The main source for the recommendations is the Choosing Wisely program, which actually presents over 500 recommendations (20). The program contains lists by specialty contributed by the national specialty societies. The health care services listed represent evidence-based recommendations. Each list provides information on when it is appropriate to perform the tests and conduct the procedures. To help you accomplish the task of reducing low-value care, the MacColl Center for Health Care Innovation created the Taking Action on Overuse framework (21).

Take a Long-Term Approach

The Health Care Transformation Task Force leadership published *Levers of Successful ACOs* (18). Their orientation is that we are in the process of health care transformation for the long term. With that point of view, it is important to support the vulnerable providers, evaluate potential partners, and enable the sustainable transition to a value-based health care economy. Toward those efforts, they give the following recommendations:

- Develop and maintain a strong culture
- Foster certain clinical practices
- Have available the data you need to function efficiently
- Openly assess your opportunities and correct the deficiency

ACOs in a Post–MACRA World

Now that you know how to be successful as an ACO, your planning has just begun. Still to consider is the Medicare Access and CHIP (Children's Health Insurance Program) Reauthorization Act (MACRA) of 2015 with interim and final rules from CMS being issued as we speak. Is this advantageous to ACOs? If so, what are the benefits? To start with, eligible clinicians can select from a few options that are available under Medicare Part B:

- An Advanced APM where the clinicians are qualified participants (QPs). The QPs earn a 5% Advanced APM bonus and are exempt from the Merit-based Incentive Payment System (MIPS).
- An Advanced APM where the clinicians are partial QPs, which means they do not meet the QP thresholds. They can either elect

to participate in MIPS and receive MIPS payment adjustments or elect to not participate in MIPS and not receive the Advanced APM bonus or MIPS adjustments.

- An alternative payment model (APM), but not an Advanced APM wherein clinicians must participate in the MIPS program and are subject to MIPS payment adjustments.
- A non-APM, which means clinicians can either elect to participate in MIPS payment adjustments or elect not to participate in MIPS.

A few facts to keep in mind: The MIPS payment adjustments are either bonuses or financial penalties. APMs and Advanced APMs include ACOs in the Medicare Shared Savings Program. The Advanced APMs, in general, have assumed downside risk as well as upside gain.

The advantages to ACOs if they become an Advanced APM with qualified participants are clear—more bonuses and no participation in a new program with new requirements. There are still advantages to Medicare ACOs that don't meet the Advanced APM and QP criteria. Those ACOs can earn MIPS bonuses as well as MSSP bonuses from cost savings. ACOs offer other advantages. They provide health information technology, data analytics, required quality reporting, care coordination, and other key infrastructure elements. Under MIPS, ACOs will automatically receive partial credit for clinical practice improvement activities points. The ACO naturally maintains a focus on population health, which keeps it current in the changing health care environment. Specialists, also, are advantaged by participating in ACOs. They benefit from care coordination, participating in the alternative payment models, and increasing their collaboration with primary care providers. In addition, if they participate in the two-sided models, such as Tracks 2 and 3 and Next Generation, the bonuses are even higher. It should be pointed out that the bonuses from MIPS are unclear at this point and depend on the achievement levels of other ACOs in the MIPS program.

An option open to ACOs, including Track 1 ACOs, is to have joined the Comprehensive Primary Care Plus (CPC+) program (22). Practices were chosen by CMS from certain states or regions of those states. The program was issued by CMS's Innovation Center and they stated that practices joining the CPC+ program qualify as Advanced APMs and are therefore exempt from MIPS. In addition, they qualify for the 5% APM incentive payment. Basically, ACOs joining CPC+ do not have to meet the financial risk criteria. That's a big change. Explanation of the two payment tracks and other details on CPC+ are covered in chapter 16.

We are at a critical junction in the changing health care environment. We have to choose a track, ultimately assume downside risk, elect a payment model, and decide whether to participate in MIPS. All require careful analysis of your current practice and to project your plans for the future. This book should facilitate you making the right decisions. In addition to the chapters already mentioned, other relevant discussions include

- an ACO's effective role in employee health plans (chapter 12),
- legal and compliance issues for ACOs (chapter 11),
- health management consulting for ACOs (chapter 15), and
- Bundled Payments for Care Improvement programs, which can be part of ACOs or compete with them (chapter 17).

Good luck!

REFERENCES

1. No results for "The US has the best health care system in the world." Bartleby website. http://www.Bartleby.com/cgi-bin/texis/webinator/sitesearch?Filter=colQuotation&query=the+US+has+the+best+health+care+system+in+the+world. Accessed September 23, 2017.

2. American health care: what's the problem? Council of Accountable Physician Practices website. http://accountablecaredoctors.org/american-healthcare-whats-the-problem. Published August 8, 2015. Accessed September 23, 2017.

3. Hiltzik M. The U.S. healthcare system: worst in the developed world. *Los Angeles Times.* June 17, 2014. http://www.latimes.com/business/hiltzik/la-fi-mh-the-us-healthcare-system-20140617-column.html. Accessed September 23, 2017.

4. Tu T, Muhlestein D, Kocot SL, White R. *The Impact of Accountable Care: Origins and Future of Accountable Care Organizations.* Washington, DC: Leavitt Partners/Brookings Institution; 2015. https://www.brookings.edu/wp-content/uploads/2016/06/Impact-of-Accountable-CareOrigins-052015.pdf. Accessed September 26, 2017.

5. Accountable Care Organizations. Definitive Healthcare website. www .definitivehc.com/ACOs. Accessed January 12, 2018.

6. Medicare Shared Savings Program Fast Facts: January 2018. Centers for Medicare and Medicaid Services website. https://www.cms.gov/Medicare/Medicare -Fee-for-Service-Payment/sharedsavingsprogram/Downloads/SSP-2018-Fast-Facts .pdf. Accessed on January 13, 2018.

7. Shared savings program. Centers for Medicare and Medicaid Services website. https://www.cms.gov/Medicare/Medicare-Fee-for-Service-Payment/sharedsavings program/index.html. Updated December 21, 2018. Accessed November 1, 2017.

8. Medicare Program; Medicare Shared Savings Program; Accountable Care Organizations: Pathways to Success and extreme and uncontrollable circumstances policies for performance year 2017. *Fed. Regist.* 2018;83(249):67816–68082. To be codified at 42 CFR §425. https://www.federalregister.gov/d/2018-27981. Accessed December 27, 2018.

9. Final policy, payment, and quality provisions changes to the Medicare physician fee schedule for calendar year 2019 [fact sheet]. Centers for Medicare and Medicaid Services website November 1, 2018. https://www.cms.gov/newsroom/fact -sheets/final-policy-payment-and-quality-provisions-changes-medicare-physician-fee -schedule-calendar-year. Accessed December 27, 2018.

10. Final rule creates pathways to success for the Medicare Shared Savings Program [fact sheet]. Centers for Medicare and Medicaid Services website. December 21, 2018. https://www.cms.gov/newsroom/fact-sheets/final-rule-creates -pathways-success-medicare-shared-savings-program. Accessed December 27, 2018.

11. New accountable care organization model opportunity: Medicare ACO Track 1+ model [fact sheet]. Centers for Medicare and Medicaid Services website. July 2017. https://www.cms.gov/Medicare/Medicare-Fee-for-Service-Payment /sharedsavingsprogram/Downloads/New-Accountable-Care-Organization-Model -Opportunity-Fact-Sheet.pdf. Accessed on November 5, 2017

12. Next Generation ACO model. CMS Innovation Center website. https:// innovation.cms.gov/initiatives/Next-Generation-ACO-Model. Updated August 20, 2019. Accessed on November 19, 2017

13. Gross PA, Easton M, Przezdecki E, et al. The ingredients of success in a Medicare accountable care organization. *Am J Accountable Care.* 2016;4(2):42–50.

14. Gross PA, Menacker M, Easton M, et al. Case study: how does an ACO generate savings three years in a row? *Am J Accountable Care.* 2017;5(2):27–31.

15. Berwick DM, Nolan TW, Whittington J. The triple aim: care, health, and cost. *Health Aff (Millwood).* 2008;27(3):759–769.

16. Pope GC, Kautter J. Minimum savings requirements in shared savings provider payment. *Health Econ.* 2015;21(11):1336–1347.

17. Population Health Management Collaborative essentials for implementing an ACO: 10 steps for a successful Medicare ACO [webinar]. Charlotte, NC: Premier Inc; September 15, 2017.

18. Health Care Transformation Task Force. *Levers of Successful ACOs.* Washington, DC: Health Care Transformation Task Force; 2017. www.hcttf.org /resources-tools-archive/2017/11/8/levers-of-successful-acos. Accessed on January 13, 2018.

19. Buxbaum JD, Mafi JN, Fendrick AM. Tackling low-value care: a new "top five" for purchaser action. *Health Affairs* blog. November 21, 2017. https://www .healthaffairs.org/do/10.1377/hblog20171117.664355/full/. Accessed December 4, 2017.

20. Clinician lists. Choosing Wisely website. www.choosingwisely.org/clinician -lists. Accessed December 4, 2017.

21. Taking Action on Overuse framework and change package. MacColl Center for Health Care Innovation website. www.maccollcenter.org/updates/events/taking -action-overuse-framework-and-change-package. Accessed December 4, 2017.

22. Comprehensive Primary Care Plus (CPC+) [FAQ list]. CMS Innovation Center website. August 1, 2016. https://innovation.cms.gov/Files/x/cpcplus-faqs.pdf. Accessed December 4, 2017.

TWO

Patient-Centered Medical Homes

A Key Building Block for Accountable Care Organizations

JOSHUA BENNETT

Recognition as a patient-centered medical home (PCMH) by the National Committee for Quality Assurance (NCQA), we feel, is a critical ingredient of achieving success as an accountable care organization (ACO). Consequently, it is the second chapter of this book. Dr. Joshua Bennett, who trains physician practices to become NCQA-recognized as PCMHs, discusses the pros and cons of certification and the chances of it improving a physician's practice and your ACO.

Introduction

Most people building accountable care organizations agree that having primary care practices that adhere to the principles, characteristics, and cultures of patient-centered medical homes greatly facilitates the financial and clinical success of their ACOs. Before we review how the PCMH concepts came into general acceptance, the resources required for you to create a PCMH, and the organizations that now recognize or accredit PCMHs, let us first discuss why they are essential to the formation and success of the your ACO.

The Patient-Centered Medical Home's Contribution to the Success of an ACO

There's a reason why the title of this chapter includes the phrase "key building block of the accountable care organization." Without the principles and functionality of PCMH practices incorporated into an ACO, the clinical and financial success of the organization is in doubt. The PCMH has patient-clinic coordination as a key function, which leads to decreased duplicate testing of patients at different sites within the ACO. Your patients can move between sites of care seamlessly, guided by your PCMH staff. This allows for greater communication between primary care and your referral network of specialists. PCMH staff continuously oversee patients' activities when they are not at the practice to ensure that they are getting the right care in the right setting at the right time. In addition, by sending your patients to the highest quality and most cost-efficient specialists, your PCMH can decrease medical costs to the ACO. Patients do not get "lost" in the system having to fend for themselves or, as a result, make choices not in their best clinical interest or the interest of your ACO. Having a system where patients can be easily seen within days of hospital discharge also contributes to lower readmission rates for the overall organization. By having PCMH staff know when your patients are admitted and discharged from an acute hospital stay, they can arrange for follow-up visits usually within seven days of discharge to prevent clinical complications from occurring and resulting in readmissions.

Access to Care

In addition, increased access to care is a critical function of the PCMH in its contribution to the success of your ACO. Presently, many practices go day after day with filled or double booked appointments and no room to add patients for acute problems. Feeling frustrated, patients may resort to going to the local emergency department, incurring a huge bill, and being cared for by a clinician not familiar with their clinical history. This leads to unnecessary admissions or, at the very least, expensive testing. If they get sent home, they are told by the emergency department physician to "follow up with your primary care physician" without contacting anyone directly to help schedule a follow-up appointment. In the PCMH and ACO environment, this whole encounter may not even happen since the PCMH is designed to have available appointments. If the encounter does occur, the emergency department can now either access the PCMH's appointment system or notify your practice that the patient was seen and to be aware that they need to follow up. In the highly functioning PCMH, the practice is "always on" and available to the patient for acute problems that may arise, thus preventing patient frustration and unnecessary visits to the emergency department.

Some ACOs have established urgent care centers that coordinate with PCMHs for after-hours care, which keeps patients from unnecessary emergency department trips. The urgent care centers may have access to the PCMH's electronic medical records so they can document the visit for the patient's primary care practitioner to see the next day, or they have established a fax connection to send the records to the PCMH after the urgent care visit.

Nurse Care Managers

Patient-centered medical homes are also the center of care management for your ACO. Nurse care managers can be imbedded within the PCMH to assist with the coordination of care and ensure that the high-risk patients do not get lost but are proactively steered back into the PCMH when it appears that they need medical attention, before they seek out the local emergency department. The nurse care managers can also see your patient panel along with the primary care provider so that the patients have a "face" to associate with those frequent telephone calls. This develops additional patient rapport with the nurse care manager so that the patients are more likely to contact them before they go somewhere else in the health care system.

Generally, each nurse care manager can have a panel of approximately 100 to 150 patients, depending on the payer mix (the more average-risk Medicare patients that are followed, the fewer complex high-risk patients that can be followed in the panel). Effective nurse care managers can easily and greatly contribute to improving the patient experience and decrease the number of visits to the emergency department and admissions to the hospital, which should lead to improved care and decreased overall costs for the ACO. In addition, nurses provide the support patients need to feel that someone else "cares" about their medical condition. All these changes improve compliance by your patients. They will follow clinical instructions better from the nurse managers and the primary care physicians, which further decreases the costs to your ACO that occurs from noncompliance with medical regimens.

Several recent studies reinforce the role of the PCMH in reducing emergency department visits and hospitalizations. The Geisinger Health System published an article in 2015 where nurse care managers imbedded in the system's PCMHs reduced total cost savings by 7.9% over a 90-month period, along with a 19% reduction in acute inpatient care (1). The Michigan Blue Cross Blue Shield Physician Group Incentive Program in 2015 demonstrated PCMH practices decreased total spending per member per month by four dollars more than control practices (a 1.1% difference) (2). The Pennsylvania Chronic Care Initiative, from 2007 to 2012, found after three years that participating PCMHs lowered all-cause hospitalizations by 1.7 admissions per 1,000 patients per month, all-cause emergency department visits by 4.7 visits per 1,000 patients per month, and ambulatory visits for specialists by 17.3 visits per 1,000 patients per month (3). These studies demonstrate a contribution by the PCMH's nurse manager to the ACO's financial success and illustrate the improvement in the care given to their patients.

Quality Outcomes

Improved clinical quality outcomes in your PCMH will also contribute to the success of your ACO. The Medicare Shared Savings Program (MSSP) is the incentive program where an ACO contracts with the Centers for Medicare and Medicaid Services to take on risk for a defined Medicare population. Those ACOs with high-functioning PCMHs have shown financial and quality metric success, especially when grouped together as a collaborative (4). If the participating ACO does not meet the 33 quality metric benchmarks (even though it meets financial benchmarks), it will have its shared savings reduced significantly. The PCMH, with its proactive approach to preventive care measures, adds greatly to meeting most of the quality metrics that MSSP requires. Most PC-MHs can generate reports using their electronic health records to find the "care gaps" of patients who have not received the recommended preventive medicine services. They then can notify their patients with gaps to make appointments to get those gaps filled, thereby increasing the score of completed preventive services.

Many commercial shared savings contracts also have Healthcare Effectiveness Data and Information Set (HEDIS) measures required to obtain shared savings. The PCMH practices are primarily responsible for ensuring that these HEDIS measures are completed. Compliance becomes critical to receiving bonus money from a shared savings contract with an insurer. While additional studies are still needed for confirmation, the need for effective PCMH practices within your ACO is essential to facilitate successful implementation of the HEDIS quality measures.

Physician Engagement

One of the challenges faced by ACOs is physician engagement and acceptance of the PCMH concepts and acclimation to the ACO culture. Financial incentives have been a primary way to improve acceptance by the practitioner. Many insurers across the country are reimbursing primary care practices for care management activities of specifically identified patient groups or for its entire insured population. The financial incentives start at five dollars per member per month and go upward from there.

In addition, the Medicare Access and CHIP Reauthorization Act of 2015 (MACRA) streamlined many quality programs under the new Merit-based Incentive Payments System (MIPS). MIPS will give bonus payments to providers for participation in eligible alternative payment models, such as eligible accountable care organizations. The implementation of MACRA is ongoing. Briefly, though, MIPS consists of four reporting areas: quality, promoting interoperability, improvement activities, and cost (5).

If your primary care practice is recognized or certified as a PCMH, then the improvement activities (presently 15% of the MIPS) are given automatic credit for the practice. The first reporting requirements were for 2017 and had to be reported by March 2018 to be eligible for a payment increase or reduction in 2019. Giving practitioners "auto credit" for a portion of the MIPS may give them incentive to transform their practices into PCMHs and then join the ACO, which would serve as an eligible alternative payment model.

Ideally you can start to appreciate the critical role PCMHs play in the success of an ACO from several different aspects. Let us now discuss the "birth" and details of the PCMH to gain a deeper understanding of their crucial role in the operations of an ACO.

Background and Development of the Patient-Centered Medical Home

Much has been written about the concept of a medical home since it was first introduced in 1967 by the American Academy of Pediatrics as a single site to store medical records of children with special health care needs (6). Over the following 40 years, numerous national discussions, debates, and proposals took place, further defining the concept. Numerous national groups—such as the North American Primary Care Research Group, the Society for Medical Decision Making, and the federal Agency for Health Care Policy and Research (now known as the Agency for Healthcare Research and Quality)—were all formed during this time. Following these groups' formations and research, numerous practice models were proposed in the late 1990s and early 2000s. In 2004, the *Annals of Family Medicine* published the final report of the Future of Family Medicine project where it stated that every American should have a personal medical home (7). The multiple proposals and models finally led four major primary care organizations—the American Academy of Family Physicians, the American Academy of Pediatrics, the American Osteopathic Association, and the American College of Physicians—to define and publish the "joint principles of the patient-centered medical home" in 2007 (8):

  o A *personal physician* who guides a team to achieve
    comprehensive, coordinated, and continuous patient care

- *Whole person orientation* through which the PCMH team coordinates aspects of a patient's care across every stage of life
- *Coordinated and/or integrated care* across the entire health care system (including specialty care as well as hospital and community-based services) that is facilitated by appropriate health information technologies, such as the electronic health records
- *Quality and safety commitment* supported by evidence-based medicine and clinical decision-support tools
- *Enhanced access to care* achieved through open scheduling, after-hours access, and improved communication between patients and providers

These were not the first principles to define how a primary care practice should function, however. In 1994, Barbara Starfield defined the "four pillars of primary care" as access to first-contact care, longitudinal continuity of care, comprehensiveness of care, and coordination of care across the other parts of the health care system (9). In 2000, the Institute of Medicine's report *Crossing the Quality Chasm* (10) became a stimulus to continue to define the principles of the patient-centered medical home. In addition, poor communication in the system and recognition of a lack of coordination between sites of care highlighted a critical safety issue in the delivery of care. During the remainder of that decade, both independent and employed family practices of varying sizes attempted to create an improved functioning medical home that focused on clinical quality, gave the patient a more meaningful experience, and relieved the pressure of the primary care physician to generate high volumes of patient visits.

Then, in 2010, the Patient Protection and Affordable Care Act (a.k.a. "Obamacare") was approved and included provisions for the encouragement and development of the medical home. It has since continued to evolve into a model of care to the point where several national organizations offer accreditation, certification, or recognition of primary care and specialty care practices to become a patient-centered medial home. To support this evolution, many states and/or health insurers now offer financial incentives for attaining such status.

In 2014, Bodenheimer et al. described the 10 building blocks of high-performing primary care practices, which incorporate Starfield's pillars, the joint principles, and PCMH recognition standards (11). They are listed in temporal order as follows:

1. Engaged leadership, creating a practice-wide vision with concrete goals and objectives
2. Data-driven improvement using computer-based technology
3. Empanelment of each patient to a care team
4. Team-based care
5. Patient-team partnership providing a framework for self-management support
6. Population management
7. Continuity of care
8. Prompt access to care
9. Comprehensiveness and care coordination
10. Template of the future requiring payment reform to reimburse for value not volume

While this methodology provided a general operational road map for practices (especially smaller practices), no significant research has yet been performed to assess whether using these building blocks in this order leads to improvement in clinical outcomes or patient and provider satisfaction.

Current Medical Home Certifying Organizations

Although Starfield's pillars of primary care and the joint principles described the critical goals of a primary care practice, they did not give specific guidance on how to operationalize the goals in a practice setting. Subsequently, the National Committee for Quality Assurance (NCQA) developed a set of standards, which has, over the last 10 years, become the overwhelming choice of primary care practices to become "recognized" or certified (12). NCQA had its roots in creating standards for PCMHs in its work on accreditation of health plans in the early 1990s. It became the dominant purveyor of health plan standards over the next 20-plus years. Using a similar process for developing the health plan standards, it brought together a large committee of experts from all stakeholder groups involved in primary care. They developed standards based on the format it used for health plan accreditation. Compliance with these standards permitted a primary care practice to become recognized. In turn, this led several other entities to create their own sets of standards all based on the joint principles in some fashion. There are now four major organizations that recognize or accredit primary care practices as medical homes:

National Committee for Quality Assurance
Utilization Review Accreditation Commission
The Joint Commission, in conjunction with its ambulatory care
    accreditation
Accreditation Association for Ambulatory Health Care

In response to the multiple offerings by entities of accreditation or recognition for PCMH, the same four organizations that developed the joint principles also developed 13 guidelines for PCMH recognition and accreditation programs in 2011 (13):

1. Incorporate the joint principles of the PCMH.

2. Address the complete scope of primary care services.

3. Ensure the incorporation of patient and family-centered care emphasizing engagement of patients, their families, and their caregivers.

4. Engage multiple stakeholders in the development and implementation of the program.

5. Align standards, elements, characteristics, and/or measures with meaningful use requirements.

6. Identify essential standards, elements, and characteristics.

7. Address the core concept of continuous improvement that is central to the PCMH model.

8. Allow for innovative ideas.

9. Care coordination within the medical neighborhood.

10. Clearly identify PCMH recognition or accreditation requirements for training programs.

11. Ensure transparency in program structure and scoring.

12. Apply reasonable documentation/data collection requirements.

13. Conduct evaluations of the program's effectiveness and implement improvements over time.

At this time, all four entities with PCMH standards have essentially met the majority of these 13 standards. This has led to core standards that are common to all four of the entities reviewing primary care practices for PCMH. Thus, over the course of 40 years, the health system has gone from a fuzzy concept of a site storing medical records for a specific category of pediatric patients to formal and consistent standards and principles for labeling a primary care practice as a PCMH for all age groups.

Resources Required for a Patient-Centered Medical Home and Financial Challenges for the Accountable Care Organization

One of the largest challenges facing a primary care practice and your ACO leadership in transforming to a recognized PCMH is what it will take in terms of financial and personnel commitment. Numerous financial studies have been performed. They vary greatly in terms of costs per provider. Halladay et al., in an article in the *Journal of the American Board of Family Medicine* (14), studied practices ranging in size from 2.5 providers to 10.5 providers. They had a wide range of payer mixes (from 7% to 43% Medicaid). They found that the average cost to become a level 3 PCMH (by NCQA 2011 standards) ranged from $11,453 to $15,977 per practice. These costs reflected new work required to prepare the application and to implement the key activities required by the PCMH standards. The practices' staffs and application authors concluded that the cost was worth the effort and that the practices all performed more efficiently after attaining the recognition.

From a practical standpoint, you as an ACO leader want to know what actually is needed to attain recognition or accreditation as a PCMH. The following is a short checklist for you. The effort and cost of each depends on the size of each practice and any affiliation with a hospital system or other private practices within your ACO. You should also consider resources you already have in place.

Electronic Health Records

Some large multispecialty groups report spending up to $30,000 per provider on ongoing information technology expenses (15). However, many smaller practices have "homegrown" systems or local/regional IT software for their electronic health records (EHRs) with total costs less than $20,000 (15). At this point in time, having a software system is almost required to perform the tasks specified by most PCMH standards. In addition, "meaningful use" standards for electronic health records, and later incarnations of what that means in relation to added reimbursement, require IT functionality that most of the PCMH standards address as well.

This is a challenge that you and most ACOs must face since many individual practices do not have the financial resources to undertake this effort. Many ACOs have provided EHRs for their provider network and integrated them into the hospital system to provide almost seamless communication between the two sites of care. The EHR is a critical piece of care coordination in highly functioning ACOs. It allows almost instantaneous information sharing between a PCMH and other sites of care, which decreases duplication of testing and services and improves communication between all sites of care, including the emergency departments of participating hospitals. The EHR allows for reporting of care gaps as noted above. It's a tool to improve HEDIS scores and quality scores for the ACO. It allows for improved team communication within the PCMH and can generate reminders for staff to notify patients who have not been seen by the practice.

Personnel Needs

A well-researched article by Sinsky et al. made the recommendation of a ratio of two to three clinical assistants (medical assistants or nurses) for each full-time equivalent physician (16). The most effective staffing model was "2 plus 1" where two medical assistants or nurses handle patient flow, the extended rooming process, and EHR information management, including visit note documentation. One clinical assistant staffs the phones, works the patient registry, and provides care coordination and care management. The additional staff salaries are more than covered by the increased efficiencies and volume of visits that each provider can see.

In addition, many practices have pulled the "plus 1" staff person out and centralized that function into one or more staff performing those functions, creating even more efficiencies with a larger practice (more than five to seven providers). If the ACO is responsible for staffing the practices, you will need to assess each practice and the staffing assigned to each site. Enough staffing is possibly the greatest issue that most primary care practices have to solve. Your ACO leadership has to address this concern fairly, logically, and on sound business models.

Space and Exam Area Modifications or Renovations

This obviously can vary with each practice. Most practices do not extensively renovate until they add providers or move locations due to the cost involved. A large majority of practices have modified workflows to accommodate the present facility floor plan. By forming dedicated teams in the "2 plus 1" staffing model and keeping that team as close to the physical space available as possible, these practices have been able to transform into PCMHs without significant facility modifications. However, the practices that have already modified their workstations into team "pod" areas appear to have the easiest time transforming their practices, increasing work efficiencies, and having more satisfied staff and providers. This presents challenges to the ACO leadership with primary care practitioners wishing to modify their practice spaces at possibly great cost. Again, most practices across the country do not modify their spaces until they need to add additional practitioners due to increased patient panel sizes.

Additional Optional Resources

For those practices with financial resources available from themselves, an affiliated hospital, insurer, or ACO, they may be able to hire patient navigators/facilitators, social workers, behavioral health specialists, or health coaches/nutritionists. These positions, in general, are not revenue-generating except for the behavioral health specialists. The practice would need to financially justify each of those positions to your ACO leadership if the ACO is decides to hire them.

Policies and Protocols Required for PCMH Transformation

One of the areas where primary care practices struggle is developing good policy and procedure documents for the primary care practice staff to follow and affect change toward a PCMH culture. All of the four entities listed earlier that accredit or recognize PCMH practices require a set of documents by which the staff is guided toward PCMH standards and principles. The practice should undergo this task with the understanding that the procedures and policies written should serve as the guidelines for how the practice is run on a daily basis. A review of the entire set of policies and procedures should take place on a yearly basis to ensure that what is written down is actually occurring within the work flows of the practice.

Basic Documentation Required for Patient-Centered Medical Homes

Many ACOs have centralized the documentation process by assigning a project manager to coordinate all the primary care practices into adopting a set of similar policies and procedures. The documents are used for the day-to-day functioning of the practice and to orient new hires. Many primary care practices assign an internal staff person to this role, while some ACOs hire an outside consultant with PCMH experience to assist the practice staff in writing and implementing the policies. Suggestions for initial policies and procedures are based on what is useful for a practice beginning the transformation journey. The documents are based on the widely used NCQA 2017 standards (17). Additional suggestions for processes to document can be found in any of the standards published by the other three entities reviewing PCMHs, but a practice should cover several of the following major areas initially.

Team-Based Care

The first area is how the practice is organized into team-based care. Organizing the practice into teams supports efficiency and decreases the chance of duplicative work and services. Communication among team members is critical for patient care and involvement. Many of these policies can be written centrally by an ACO staff member for use in all of the ACO's practices. This approach will facilitate staffing and centralized quality reporting. Here is a list of policies and procedures with questions to consider:

Organization structure. Who is in charge of the practice? How is the practice organized into teams? What does the practice's overall structure look like?

Job descriptions. All practice staff should have a detailed job description that includes role, skills required, responsibilities, fit into the team concept, training required, licenses required, physical requirements, goals, and objectives. Identify frequency of evaluation as well.

Practice participation in outside initiatives such as ACO activities or Medicare reporting. How is this accomplished and reported? What outcomes are reported? Who is responsible for reporting? How often are reports generated? Where are they located?

Patient involvement in the practice. How are patients involved in the quality activities of the practice? Is there a patient advisory council? Can they be members of a board of directors? How do they get selected? Is there a charter for the council or board?

Team communication. Is there a daily huddle? How does it work? How do team members communicate patient information to each other?

Quality improvement activities of the practice. How are quality activities organized? Is all staff involved with the practice's quality activities? Who is in charge of those activities and how do they get reported to internal and external entities?

Information to patients. How does the practice give information to the patients? Is there an orientation packet? What does it include? Is there a website for the practice? How do patients access it?

Managing and Understanding the Practice's Patients

In order to deliver the highest quality care, a practice needs to know the needs of its patient population and provide patient materials to increase patient engagement. Using evidence-based guidelines is also essential for consistent, high-quality care. The ACO as an entity may decide to adopt nationally accepted guidelines, or its clinicians may generate new ones based on local care delivery practices. The ACO may keep a central repository of community resources and generate all of the patient materials. There are several policies that can be included:

Performing a comprehensive patient assessment. How does the practice collect data on family history, past medical history, behavioral health history, social and cultural needs, communication with the patient, risky behaviors, activities of daily living, social determinants of health, developmental screens for pediatric patients, advance care planning, depression and behavioral health screening, and oral health screening? How does it perform medication reconciliation?

Patient materials. Does the practice use easy-to-understand health education material, and how does it make sure the patient receives it? Does the practice use clinical decision support materials, and how does the patient use them?

Evidence-based guidelines. Does the practice use them? Which ones are implemented into the workflow of the practice? Do the patients know evidence-based guidelines are being used by the practice?

Community resources. Does the practice use and access community resources for their patients? Which ones are used? How does the practice evaluate which resources are useful for the patient? Are there patient education classes available and which ones? Does the practice have a relationship with a school/intervention agency in the community?

How does this work? Does the practice utilize case conferences outside the practice?

Patient Access and Continuity of Care

This is an area critical to patient satisfaction and engagement. It shows how the PCMH can make your ACO more successful. Your staffing and resources are critical to ensuring adequate access. Basic guidelines for access are as follows:

Access to the practice. How does the practice assess whether access is adequate? How are same-day appointments handled? How are different types of patient visits defined? How are patients handled after hours and weekends? Are there patient hours outside of the usual 8:00 a.m. to 5:00 p.m. work schedule? How do the patients contact the practice during and after hours? How are the contacts handled? Can the patient use a web portal to contact the practice? How are these handled? Are alternative appointments (such as video, email, etc.) available, and how are these handled?

Assigning patients to providers. How is this handled? Is it done during patient orientation? Is the goal for the patient to see their assigned primary care provider as much as possible? Is there a target goal for this? How do other providers access patient information when they are covering the practice? Does the practice have a process to review the number of patients assigned to each clinician? Does the practice receive reports of paneled patients from outside entities, and what does it do with those?

Care Management

This is an area in which many practices are just beginning to implement across the country. Assistance is offered by health plans and the practices' parent hospital systems. ACOs, as mentioned earlier, may be responsible for assigning care managers to each practice. They also establish criteria for enrolling patients and deciding levels of patient panels each care manager can handle.

Identifying patients. The major policy you should include is identifying patients for care management. What are the criteria the practice uses for finding those patients that require additional care management by a nurse or other staff member? How does it develop a care plan for each of those identified? What is the size of the care manager's patient panel? What does the care plan include? How does it measure the success of the care management program?

Care Coordination and Transitions of Care

One of the key issues with the health care system in the United States is the lack of coordination of care between sites of care. This leads to duplication of testing and services, patient errors, patient injury, and delay in getting needed clinical services. The PCMH should be the center of coordinating care for each patient in your ACO and include three coordinating policies in its plan:

Tracking laboratory and imaging studies. Your practice should describe in detail its process for ordering, tracking, and recording both laboratory and imaging studies from the practice. A "close the loop" process should ensure that all laboratory and imaging studies ordered are performed and your ordering provider reviews the results and acts upon them in a timely fashion. There should be a process by which abnormal results are flagged and brought promptly to the attention of the ordering provider. Timely notification of both normal and abnormal results should be given to the patients. This policy should also include newborn screening tests if the practice sees newborns and pediatric patients. The practice should have a policy and procedure for reviewing testing to assess if over- or underutilization is occurring.

Tracking of referrals to specialists. A policy should define what information you send to the specialist for a consultation, the clinical question that is being asked, the patient's demographic and insurance information, and a time frame for a documented response. The practice should have a process to track all referrals and ensure that they are completed in a reasonable time frame. The provider should review the report and act on it accordingly. A documented relationship should be established with behavioral health professionals to facilitate the easy referral of potentially challenging mental health patient issues. Documented relationships or comanagement agreements between the practice and specialists should also be described. A process to assess to whom the practice refers patients should be described. National "report cards" or other means should be used to assess the specialists.

Unplanned visits to the emergency department/hospital. Your practice should describe what it does for these visits and how it is made aware in a timely fashion that they have occurred. Discharging patients from these settings should have a defined process for follow-up with the referring practice in a timely fashion. The process should be tracked to ensure that follow-ups are occurring within established time frames. Arrangements for patients to be seen at other sites, such as urgent care centers, should be described. Access to the practice's electronic health record should be made available to the urgent care centers. A method to obtain discharge summaries from hospitalized patients should be described.

Quality Improvement and Measurement

Without measuring quality outcomes, the success of the PCMH, and ultimately your ACO, can be questioned. If you don't measure it, you can't improve it. Highly functioning PCMH practices report their quality and cost metrics to their providers (and to the ACO) at least on a monthly basis. This reporting provides real-time feedback on the practice's performance. ACOs are dependent on their PCMHs to deliver improvement in HEDIS scores and other preventive clinical services to fulfill their shared savings contracts.

Quality measures. The policy should include what is measured, how data is collected, and what is done with the results. A key metric is reviewing the availability of all appointment types and how they are filled and then reported to staff and providers. How the practice collects and reports patient satisfaction surveys to the practice staff is critical. Identification of vulnerable populations within the practice is important to assess for disparity of care for those populations. Goals or benchmarks for the quality metrics should be defined. The results should be measured against the benchmarks and reported to the providers and staff on a regular basis. A process should be developed to report all quality measures to the practice's patients, your ACO, and external entities.

In addition to these policies and procedures, the four entities reviewing practices for PCMH standards require numerous clinical and administrative reports to support those policies. These reports should be concise, easily interpreted, and include the time frame in which the data were collected. They also should be relevant to the running of the practice and for patient care improvement. Many ACOs have centralized the reporting function that generates reports by practice and practitioner to assist them in closing care gaps and assessing their clinical efficiencies. Taking time to precisely document what the practice and your ACO is reporting will give the reviewing entities evidence that the practice is embracing the principles of the patient-centered medical home.

If all of the requirements in the above six areas sound a little overwhelming and intimidating, they are. If you do all of the above, however, you should qualify for recognition by NCQA standards.

The Patient-Centered Medical Home Culture as Part of the Accountable Care Organization Culture

In many of the country's primary care practices and hospital systems, the culture is still "provider centric." That is, all the workflow processes and decisions are made with the providers as the focus: Schedules are made around the provider's wishes. Patients have to coordinate their own care, and many are double-booked most days. The practice finds out weeks later that their patients were in the emergency department or hospitalized, and the patients get lost in the system as a result. It is believed that great quality care is delivered because the providers are well trained.

Most of the time, however, providers still feel like they are on a treadmill trying to keep up with the ever-growing demands of seeing patients. They are filling out paper work trying to recall all the preventive care services a patient requires, and sending off referrals and lab and imaging requests while not remembering to check to see if requests have been returned.

Your practice's staff feel like they are overextended trying to room patients, call back test results to patients, and keep their provider happy at all times.

All of these problems are addressed by PCMH principles, organization, and culture. In highly functioning PCMH practices and ACOs, there is a proactive or "patient-centered" approach always present. Patients are called ahead of their scheduled appointments for reminders. Testing takes place before the visit so the results are available at the time of the visit. This practice eliminates an after-visit telephone call to the patient with the results. In addition, the provider has an excellent opportunity to discuss test results face-to-face with the patient and affect behavioral change if necessary. All aspects of the practice are measured constantly to look for areas of improvement from both the patient- and practice-side of workflows. Sufficient same-day appointments are a standard feature of the PCMH to allow adequate time for patients with acute clinical problems to be seen at the practice rather than the emergency department.

Patients sick enough to be seen in the emergency department or admitted to the hospital after hours are known by the practice since it has set up a notification system with the local hospitals. A follow-up post-hospitalization appointment is set up by the practice usually within five to seven days of discharge to prevent a readmission. Medication lists are constantly reconciled no matter where the patient is. Team members work to the "top of their license" in this culture. That is, physicians are not filling out paper work, which a front office person could be doing. Nurses are providing education to the patients instead of performing vital signs. The medical assistants are rooming patients, performing medication reconciliation, taking vital signs, recording the present complaint, and returning calls to patients. In some practices, medical assistants act as "scribes" to the providers to facilitate and enhance the patient-physician interaction instead of the physician having their head buried in the computer screen during the patient visit. One can see that all of these characteristics are essential to the efficiency of the overall workings of your ACO and to improve its patient satisfaction, quality outcomes, and financial bottom line.

In a nationwide study, the Peterson Center on Healthcare and Stanford University's Clinical Excellence Research Center set out to find high-performing primary care providers through an analysis that identified primary care practices delivering higher quality care at lower total annual cost (18). They found 11 frontline primary care practices across the country that all had 10 characteristics of the PCMH culture in common:

1. *These practices were "always on."* Patients knew that their care teams were always available and they would be able to reach someone that would help them quickly, whether or not the practice was closed.

2. *The physicians adhered to quality guidelines and chose tests and treatments wisely.* They had systems that ensured patients received evidence-based care yet conserved resources by tailoring care to align with the needs and values of their patients.

3. *They treated patient complaints as gold.* These were regarded as valuable as compliments, and staff took every opportunity to encourage patient feedback to improve the patient experience.

4. *They insourced, rather than outsourced, some needed tests and procedures.* The providers did as much as they could clinically and safely before referring patients out to specialists. These included skin biopsies, joint injections, suturing, and insulin initiation.

5. *They stayed close to their patients after referring them to specialists.* The practices chose specialists they could work closely with and whom they trusted to return their patients to their care after the specialist had finished with them. In some cases, they comanaged patients with the specialists so they could keep medication and problem lists up to date.

6. *They closed the loop with patients.* They actively followed up to make sure patients were seen by them soon after hospital discharge or seen by a specialist.

7. *They maximized the abilities of staff members.* This consisted of all staff working at the "top of their licenses" as noted earlier.

8. *They worked in "hived workstations."* The care team worked side by side in an open "bullpen" environment that enhanced continuous communication among both clinical and nonclinical staff.

9. *They balanced compensation.* Physicians were paid not based just on volume but also from at least one of the following: quality of care, patient experience, resource utilization, and contribution to practice-wide improvement activities.

10. *They invested in people, not space and equipment.* They rented modest offices. They invested in equipment if it allowed them to provide care more cost-effectively. They had at least two staff for every provider seeing patients and usually had three for one provider.

These 10 characteristics all led to benefiting the ACO. More satisfied practitioners and patients led to better perceptions that the ACO was actually improving their clinical care and the overall patient experience. The successful ACOs have begun to master this patient-centered culture and have been the "winners" so far with the Medicare Shared Savings Program. By adopting the majority of the characteristics above, your ACO and PCMHs will improve your patient experiences, clinical quality outcomes, staff and provider experiences, and financial outcomes.

Accreditation and Recognition Programs Available for the Primary Care Practice

As mentioned earlier, four entities presently either accredit or recognize primary care practices as being a patient-centered medical home. The National Committee for Quality Assurance is the dominant player in recognizing primary care practices, with over 13,000 sites and 67,000 practitioners being recognized as of early 2019 (19). However, the Utilization Review Accreditation Commission (URAC), The Joint Commission, and the Accreditation Association for Ambulatory Health Care (AAAHC) all have comparable standards and requirements and make up approximately 25% of the country's practices that have accreditation or certification (20).

The Medical Group Management Association produced a tool to compare all four of these entities' recognition/accreditation programs to the "Guidelines for the Patient-Centered Home Recognition and Accreditation Programs" published by the American Academy of Family Physicians, the American Academy of Pediatrics, the American Osteopathic Association, and the Advisory Committee on Immunization Practices (20). This tool reveals that all entities do meet the majority of these guidelines, and which program a practice chooses for recognition, certification, or accreditation may depend on the practice's needs and particular situation. For example, a hospital-based practice may choose The Joint Commission for accreditation because its parent hospital uses The Joint Commission for its hospital and ambulatory accreditation survey and can "piggy back" on that survey for no additional cost. Table 2.1 summarizes the main areas of focus for the four entities.

Table 2.1. Standards comparison of the four major patient-centered medical home accrediting entities

National Committee for Quality Assurance	Utilization Review Accreditation Commission	The Joint Commission	Accreditation Association for Ambulatory Health Care
Six standards:	Seven modules:	Five operational characteristics:	Five standards:
1. Team-based care and practice organization	1. Core quality care management	1. Patient-centered care	1. Relationship, communication, understanding, and collaboration
2. Knowing and managing your patients	2. Patient-centered operations management	2. Comprehensive care	2. Accessibility
3. Patient-centered access and continuity	3. Access and communication	3. Coordinate care	3. Comprehensiveness of care
4. Care management and support	4. Testing and referrals	4. Superb access to care	4. Continuity of care
5. Care coordination and care transitions	5. Care management and coordination	5. System-based approach to quality and safety	5. Quality
6. Performance measurement and quality improvement	6. Advance electronic capability and patient registry		
	7. Quality performance reporting and improvement		

It is apparent that all four entities cover the same 13 guidelines with the slight exception of AAAHC and The Joint Commission on guideline 5, which is aligning with meaningful use requirements. The other major difference among these entities' standards is AAAHC, URAC, and The Joint Commission use an on-site survey. NCQA now uses a collaborative method for its 2017 standards where the NCQA reviewer meets by telephone and virtually over three separate occasions in several hour sessions with the practice staff to review the documents submitted in support of the practice's application. The reviewer notes those documents requiring modification and makes a request to have them resubmitted at the next telephone conference. This has taken the place of the practices submitting all documents to a website where the NCQA reviewer would review and score them. Of note is the fact that NCQA also has a set of standards for a specialty practice-based PCMH. It is referred to as patient-centered specialty practice recognition. In addition, there is a subset of standards for oncology: the oncology medical home recognition. The standards are based on the PCMH standards but oriented to the specialists' perspective. The standards and how to apply for recognition is available on the NCQA website on the PCMH Recognition Process page (21).

Finally, the cost of each entity's program varies as well:

- The average fee for medical home accreditation by AAAHC ranges from $4,500 to $26,000.
- The Joint Commission's primary care medical home certification incurs no extra cost for organizations that receive its ambulatory accreditation survey. A separate survey can run from a three-year total fee of $9,000 to $27,000 based on patient volume and number of sites.
- URAC's fee can range from $3,500 to $14,000 determined by the number of reviewers and number of on-site days to survey the practice sites.
- NCQA's fees are based on the number of providers in the practice. The fee is $550 for up to 12 providers. For 12–50 providers, the fee is $6,600, and for more than 50 providers, the fee is $6,600 plus $10 per provider over 50.

These fees are examples of each entity's information as of 2018. Please check each entity's website for updated fees when you apply.

Key Pathways for Creating a Successful ACO

In conclusion, it is apparent that the patient-centered medical home concept has gone through a great deal of change and modifications since its inception. While over 14,000 practices have been designated as PCMHs, a great deal more are still lacking that designation. Several well-known organizations certify, accredit, and recognize primary care practices as PCMHs. All are similar in their requirements.

The PCMH has been shown to be a key building block of an ACO. The PCMH provides numerous opportunities for improving quality and financial efficiencies as well as patient and provider satisfaction. Yet, more research needs to be performed to solidify the PCMH's primary position as the model for the center of the future health care delivery system. Many challenges still remain, but it appears that the health care system is slowly moving in the correct direction—toward value-based rather than volume-based medical care. Adapting the Clinical Excellence Research Center's 10 points of highly performing primary care organizations will further assure your success as an ACO.

For you, the PCMH is a ready way to participate in the transformation of health care and be successful. It will show you how to provide team-based coordinated care, facilitate access, improve the patient and physician experience, ensure quality and safety, develop better care management tools, and significantly reduce the cost of care. Then you will survive in the evolving shift to value-based care.

REFERENCES
    1. Maeng DD, Khan N, Tomcavage J, Graf TR, Davis DE, Steele GD. Reduced acute inpatient care was largest savings component of Geisinger Health System's patient-centered medical home. *Health Aff (Millwood)*. 2015;34(4):636–644. doi:10.1377/hlthaff.2014.0855.
    2. Lemak CH, Nahra TA, Cohen GR, et al. Michigan's fee-for-value physician incentive program reduces spending and improves quality in primary care. *Health Aff (Millwood)*. 2015;34(4):645–652. doi:10.1377/hlthaff.2014.0426.

3. Friedberg MW, Rosenthal MB, Werner RM, Volpp KG, Schneider EC. Effects of a medical home and shared savings intervention on quality and utilization of care. *JAMA Intern Med.* 2015;175(8):1362–1368. doi:10.1001/jamainternmed.2015 .2047.

4. Premier Inc. Population Health Management Collaborative, private correspondence, 2017.

5. MIPS overview. Quality Payment Program website. Centers for Medicare and Medicaid Services. http://www.qpp.cms.gov/mips/overview. Accessed March 21, 2018.

6. Sia C, Tonniges TF, Osterhus E, Taba S. History of the medical home concept. *Pediatrics.* 2004;113(5 Suppl):1473–1478.

7. Martin, JC, Avant RF, Bowman MA, et al. The Future of Family Medicine: a collaborative project of the family medicine community. *Ann Fam Med.* 2004;2(Suppl 1):S3–32.

8. Joint principles of the patient-centered medical home [news release]. American Academy of Family Physicians, American Academy of Pediatrics, American College of Physicians, American Osteopathic Association; March 2007. https://www.aafp.org /dam/AAFP/documents/practice_management/pcmh/initiatives/PCMHJoint.pdf. Accessed March 20, 2018.

9. Starfield B. Is primary care essential? *Lancet.* 1994;344(8930):1129–1133. doi:10.1016/s0140-6736(94)90634-3.

10. Institute of Medicine. *Crossing the Quality Chasm: A New Health System for the 21st Century.* Washington, DC: National Academies Press; 2000.

11. Bodenheimer T, Ghorob A, Willard-Grace R, Grumbach K. The 10 building blocks of high-performing primary care. *Ann Fam Med.* 2014;12(2):166–171. doi:10.1370/afm.1616.

12. NCQA PCMH recognition: concepts. National Committee for Quality Assurance website. https://www.ncqa.org/programs/health-care-providers-practices /patient-centered-medical-home-pcmh/pcmh-concepts. Accessed October 14, 2019.

13. Guidelines for patient-centered medical home (PCMH) recognition and accreditation program [news release]. American Academy of Family Physicians, American Academy of Pediatrics, American College of Physicians, American Osteopathic Association; February 2011. https://www.aafp.org/dam/AAFP/documents /practice_management/pcmh/initiatives/PCMHJoint2011.pdf. Accessed March 20, 2018.

14. Halladay JR, Mottus K, Reiter K, et al. The cost to successfully apply for level 3 medical home recognition. *J Am Board Fam Med.* 2016;29(1)69–77. doi:10.3122/jabfm.2016.01.150211.

15. Personal correspondence with several hospital system multispecialty groups. 2016.

16. Sinsky CA, Willard-Grace R, Schutzbank AM, Sinsky TA, Margolius D, Bodenheimer T. In search of joy in practice: a report of 23 high-functioning primary care practices. *Ann Fam Med.* 2013;11(3):272–278. doi:10.1370/afm.1531.

17. NCQA PCMH Standards and Guidelines (epub). National Committee for Quality Assurance website. http://store.ncqa.org/index.php/catalog/product/view/id /2776/s/pcmh-standards-and-guidelines-epub. Accessed October 14, 2019.

18. Identification: uncovering America's most valuable care. Peterson Center on Healthcare website. http://petersonhealthcare.org/identification-uncovering-americas -most-valuable-care. Accessed March 15, 2018.

19. Patient-centered medical home recognition. National Committee for Quality Assurance website. http://www.ncqa.org/employers/ncqa-programs-of-interest-to -employers/patient-centered-medical-home-recognition. Accessed March 20, 2019.

20. Medical Group Management Association. *The Patient Centered Medical Home Guidelines: A Tool to Compare National Programs.* Englewood, CO: MGMA; 2011. http://csimt.gov/wp-content/uploads/MGMA-PCMH-Guidelines_Tool-to -Compare-National-Programs.pdf. Accessed March 30, 2018.

21. The PCMH recognition process. National Committee for Quality Assurance website. https://www.ncqa.org/programs/health-care-providers-practices/patient -centered-medical-home-pcmh/process. Accessed March 25,2018.

THREE

Care Coordination

Initial Plans and Evolution

DENISE PATRIACO

> *Starting a care coordination program is the next most important activity you can implement to achieve success as an accountable care organization. Care coordinators are trained to assist physician practices by focusing on the high-risk patients. They help the physician with recommendations for improving the experience of care and complying with the quality measures from the Centers for Medicare and Medicaid Services or other payers. Denise Patriaco, APN, set up our care coordination program. She trained at Duke and now is the administrator running our ACO. She concludes the chapter with the keys to a successful care coordination program. Follow her recommendations carefully and yours will be a success.*

Introduction

Care coordination plays a critical role for your ACO and for all your population health programs. Many ACOs struggle to create efficient and measurable care coordination programs, however, which can significantly impact cost and satisfaction scores. One common strategy is to purchase software with risk scores and pretemplated documentation tools combined with admission-discharge-transfer (ADT) vendors. What is missing in this approach is a plan for how care coordination teams are trained, supported, monitored, and eventually evaluated. Most of the commentary and opinions in this chapter focus on my experience with an embedded care coordination model. I emphasize provider practice-level workflows and the placement of nurses and other clinical/nonclinical staff within primary care practices. Supplemental centralized coordination is used on a small scale for practices with low beneficiary counts. The evidence suggests that focusing efforts in the primary care setting will improve ACO performance (1).

Organizations that use a care coordination model with standardized and measurable interventions are associated with lower spending and improved health outcomes (2). These are high-level recommendations on how to organize and execute a care coordination program that is truly effective. As I write this, my organization was ranked number three in ACO savings nationwide. You should take from this chapter what seems to make sense within your organization.

Assessment and Evaluation for a Care Coordination Program

The initial work in creating a care coordination program is unarguably daunting and often assigned to people with little to no experience in population management or care coordination. Undoubtedly, most programs begin with thousands of patients to be "covered" by one or two nurses. In organizing and hiring staff, there are a few initial items to keep in mind during your planning.

How Many Patients Are in Your Program?

Most programs use nurse–patient ratios of 1 to 3,500, which includes about 150 patients that would be considered high risk. Keeping this ratio as small as possible while considering your case mix of patients will allow your nursing staff to make true differences in the costs and health outcomes of your population.

You will have to look at your population and determine the number of, for example, frail elderly Medicare patients versus younger, healthier commercial patients. There is no set ratio for nurses to patients; it will be unique to your population and specific care components that are unnecessarily increasing your total spend.

You must know your case mix of patients and create a plan for how specifically this ratio of nurses to patients is going to change in order to improve the health of your population as well as lower your costs.

How Many Are Elderly and/or Disabled?

As partially explained above, these are the two groups of patients that will require the most coordination time. If a total population has a large percentage of elderly or disabled, it would make sense to decrease the nurse–patient ratio.

How Large Are the Practices in Your Organization and How Much Distance Is Between Them?

While there are other items you will be considering, such as practice engagement and motivation, covering large practices first will provide you with the greatest impact on your organization because you will be covering more patients in one place. If you are planning to have staff cover more than one practice, be sure the geographical distance is realistic and manageable so that staff is not wasting too much time driving between offices.

Who Are the Internal and External Stakeholders?

Who is going to support your program with resources financially, clinically, and educationally? Meeting with all of these stakeholders, both collectively and individually, on a regular basis will provide stability and direction for your program. It is up to care coordination management to keep all stakeholders abreast of victories as well as obstacles and to enlist their support. The saying "people will support what they help create" certainly applies here.

What Type of Team Will You Need?

I have noticed that many organizations make the mistake of becoming too top-heavy. That is, there is an ample amount of management but not enough frontline staff. At minimum, you will need a manager to organize and administer the initial effort of creating and operationalizing a care coordination team. Ample care coordinators are, of course, required. But along with nurses as the coordinators, a nonlicensed staff should also be added to do the clerical and nonclinical work that is required. Examples of this nonclinical work are quality metric mining, making appointments for patients, scanning, and filing.

Data will be extremely important for you to use to gauge the progress of your overall program as well as performance of your individual providers and practices. You should hire a data analyst to create and help interpret reports on a regular basis. You should create and maintain good communication with your chief medical officer or a like physician position from the ACO management staff. That person will assist you in working with the providers on a one-on-one basis to review quality and financial data as well as influencing referrals to in-network providers.

How Will You Share Data with Other Providers and Services?

It is essential to know where your attributed members are each day in the circle of hospital to home. Patients in transition pose the greatest threat for poor health outcomes. Therefore, keeping in close contact with them during this period can save your organization significant dollars.

Obtaining an ADT feed of major hospitals, subacute facilities, and visiting nursing services, as well as obtaining your commercial payer's daily admission lists, is instrumental for effective care coordination. In addition, determining how your care team will communicate with in- and out-of-network services and providers is recommended.

Plan a Strategy

The overall initial structure of your care coordination team should reflect the targeted population's needs. Review all available data on attributed members to respond accordingly with staffing. For example, if you have a large population of diabetics that are incurring significant costs, you should be hiring care coordinators with good diabetic management experience. The diabetic coordinator will improve not only the glycemic control of the patients but also work on other comorbidities that lead to poor outcomes and high costs. If your providers feel that you are able to impact their patients in a meaningful way, you will quickly gain their support. Then they will likely be more interested in working with your team to reduce costs.

I am always going to suggest starting a program with the most qualified nurses who can perform the majority of responsibilities and tasks. A registered nurse (RN) can assess and educate patients, coordinate services, reconcile medications, and also mine and report quality metrics as needed. A medical assistant, however, cannot perform all of those functions. In the initial program launch, I suggest hiring the higher-level registered nurse to perform all aspects of care coordination and then six months to one year after program launch, expand your RN reach to patients by hiring medical assistants and clerical positions to perform the non-RN responsibilities. The purpose of hiring the RNs first is to have a complete evaluation of responsibilities; that is, have the RNs actually work those responsibilities themselves so that there is a true understanding of the time, tools, and resources needed. When all the appropriate full-time equivalent positions are hired, the management and care coordinators are able to monitor and evaluate the activities objectively and serve as a continual resource.

Once the care coordination program has been in effect for about one to two years, it will be easier for you to understand all the needs of the team, resources required, and appropriate level of staffing. It is at this point when the RN care coordinators should focus on effective and efficient patient care. Then your support staff will be in place for other necessary activities. This prevents the RN care coordinator from performing duties that take him or her away from patient care.

Care Coordination Documentation Basics

Your care coordination team should have one standard documentation tool whenever possible. Although this may not be feasible when you first begin your program, it should be a priority to get in place as soon as you are able. A standard format is the best way to pull data and other important information about your population. It is also a way to measure care coordination activity and productivity. RN positions are costly. You will need staff productivity reports to demonstrate that your nurse–patient ratios are appropriate. Also, the reports can assist you in evaluating the effectiveness of each care coordinator.

There are many vendors who will promote platforms that promise the world. Unfortunately, most come in very expensive, pretty packages with little to no usable content. Beware of purchasing expensive software in the early stages of a program. Take into account the intent of the nursing note. Is it for data mining? Is it for communication with other providers and services? Is it for something else or for all of the above? Review the care notes of other organizations and create some of your own before purchasing pretemplated software. Creating note templates is essential to ensuring that nurses are collecting the most important information each time they speak with a patient or family. It is important to standardize documentation so that it can be used to pull data.

There are certain types of note templates you will want depending on the patient situation. Examples of common note types are those for post-acute care/emergency room visits, post-subacute/rehabilitation records, and high-risk patient care.

Creating Space for and Building Relationships with Care Coordinators

Space in a primary care office is almost always limited, whether the practice is very busy or whether the physical building is big or small. When embedding care coordinators, it is best for ACO management to view the office space for themselves and have a discussion with the practice leaders on the amount of space and equipment care coordination will need. In some instances, it will be very difficult for you to convince the practice to accept the concept of a care coordinator within their practice. Those who have not worked with a care coordinator (especially, a *good* care coordinator) do not know how much they will enhance their costs, patient care, and patient satisfaction.

My organization has had care coordinators working in empty exam rooms with laptops and cellphones at times, just to get started within the practice. So care coordination management should be prepared to supply each coordinator with the minimum of a laptop, cell phone, and hot spot for Wi-Fi, but once the practice staff and providers realize the contributions of the care coordinator, they will likely give them more-suitable working space and equipment because they now view the co-ordinator as a valued team member. It cannot be stressed strongly enough that if the care coordinators do not find a way to prove their worth and become part of the culture and spirit of the practice, they will likely not be effective within that practice.

The best way to build relationships with practices is to hit the ground running and show your worth as soon as possible. One way we did this was to have the care coordinators ask each provider in the practice to give them the names of their top five patients that they worried about or would not be surprised if they were admitted to the hospital or the emergency room that day. The care coordinator immediately began working with those patients, taking the burden of worry off the back of the provider.

Another good idea is to have the care coordinator shadow each role within the practice, which is described in more detail on page 74 and in the case study on page 86. One of the biggest complaints I hear from practices who had previous care coordinators before my team is that they did not know what a care coordinator did. This statement equates to the practice not seeing or feeling the value of having a care coordinator. In this situation, the care coordinator may not last.

Once the care coordinator is in the practice for a few days, there will be multiple transitional patients to follow and bring back into the office, so the caseload will naturally increase. It is important for the care coordinator to communicate early on to the providers which patients he or she is working with and why. The care coordinator should let the providers know that they can request her help at any time. It will be the care coordinator's job to open up communication and forge relationships for quite some time.

Creating a Care Coordination Program
Choosing Candidates and Interviewing

The initial staff chosen to begin a care coordination program is quite important. This staff will be the initial face of your organization and shape your early credibility and successes. Sometimes this means hiring people with experience and other times this means hiring people who are thirsty to learn, motivated to succeed, and willing to be intensively trained.

When I interview for any position, I tell the candidate at the end of the interview, "I can teach you anything you need to learn to be successful here except the two most important factors for your success and longevity. Those two things are a work ethic and how to be nice. These two things cannot be taught; you will need to already possess these two personality traits, or you will not be happy in our organization."

Usually by the time I say this, I have a good idea of both traits because my interviews are more about having a conversation than asking pointed questions. In this setting, the candidates are relaxed, and more of their true personality is revealed.

Orientation

Many organizations think that any nurse can be an effective care coordinator. This is far from the truth. Care coordinators must be taught. It is very important to the success of any program that the *right* people are chosen for the positions and an effective, standardized education or orientation is offered. There should always be an orientation program that includes

- classroom education on the basics of value-based care,
- an introduction to the organization and its purpose,
- review of tools available for care coordination,
- review of resources,
- on-site training, and
- a buddy-system for the orientation period and afterward.

Standardizing Outreach Workflows

Standardization should be a goal for all programs. Which patients and under what circumstances the coordinators reach out to patients should be consistent. The three ways I like to divide outreach is transitional contacts, post-acute contacts, and provider referral/high-risk contacts.

Transitional Contacts

These are patients who are moving through acute care or emergency room (ER) care to home with or without visiting nursing services. Managing care transitions from the inpatient to outpatient setting is critical to improving patient outcomes and reducing costs (3). The optimal time to contact these patients and/or family is when they are *still in* the hospital if at all possible. This is more realistic for inpatients than ER patients, but depending on what your organization utilizes for ADT alerts, speaking with patients while they are in the ER is possible.

With the increased use of hospitalists, many primary care providers (PCPs) do not participate in hospital rounds for their patients anymore. It can be days before the hospitalist contacts the PCP, and sometimes the contact never occurs. About half of adults in the United States experience a medical error after a hospital discharge, and 19%–23% suffer an adverse event during inpatient to outpatient care transitions (4). This is when care coordination can become so valuable. The care coordinator should reach out to the patient to reassure them that their PCP is aware they have been hospitalized, is following along with the hospital-based care, and will be updated and ready to continue the patient's care once discharged.

The provider and the coordinator should work with the hospitalist and inpatient care managers for a seamless transition to the home settings with all durable medical equipment and follow-up visits scheduled. Once discharged, the care coordinator should contact the patient within 48 hours to ensure that the patient is aware of symptoms to report and has all medication prescribed. Again, the importance of the follow-up appointment with the PCP (and specialist when needed) should be stressed by the care coordinator.

Post-Acute Contacts

Many areas of the country are facing long Medicare lengths of stay within subacute facilities. The underlying issue here is misaligned incentives for value-based organizations and the skilled nursing facilities (SNFs). The SNF still operates largely in a fee-for-service payment system. Another serious problem with post-acute facilities is the high rate of readmissions to inpatient settings. These issues will result in significant cost increases for an ACO if not routinely monitored and addressed. Simple care coordination activities such as ongoing communication with post-acute facilities and enhanced information sharing are likely a key contributor to the lower readmissions for ACO facilitated hospitals.

The care coordinator should be used to contact the SNF at least weekly to coordinate and encourage an appropriate discharge date. The patient goals for discharge should be discussed each week and compared to exactly where the patient has progressed. Often found are lofty goals that the patient will not every achieve. For example, if a patient could not walk more than 25 feet before hospitalization, why now is the ambulation goal for discharge that the patient should walk 100 feet? The care coordinator must consistently evaluate (along with the physician) the necessity of stay within realistic parameters and maintain consistent contact with the SNF.

Provider Request versus List of High-Risk Patients

Although inconsistent with what is commonly noted in value-based literature strategies, I have never used a "high-risk" list for care coordination contacts. The reason is that these lists are often based on claim data that is three to six months outdated. The care coordination team should know when a patient is admitted to a hospital or has made an emergency room visit by using the ADT system of the ACO and by using payer reports. The admit or emergency room visit should be followed up at that time rather than waiting six months and finding out the patient was readmitted multiple times. It is important to intervene as soon as possible after an unplanned hospital visit in order to have the greatest impact on preventing another.

Because high-risk lists also use spending as a top criterion, many of the patients tend to not be candidates for care coordination. These patients are most often going through active cancer treatment or have high-cost health services like dialysis, and care coordination is not going to be able to decrease costs or optimize the patient's quality of life. These patients are most often managed by specialists who manage all of the patient's care needs—even those that are traditionally managed by the PCP.

Instead, the high-risk list is used in my organization as a second check to determine if we are missing someone who is a candidate for care coordination. Most often, what is found are patients who are receiving care in another part of the country (they moved or are "snowbirds"), have mental issues, are noncompliant/resistant with past attempts of care coordinators, have high-cost medications that cannot be changed, or are in active treatment as stated above.

To reiterate, provider requests for care coordination are picked up each day within my organization. When we first began, each care coordinator asked their assigned providers for a list of patients that they worried about being hospitalized or suffering poor health outcomes. With that list and the ADT list, the care coordination program took off.

Tools for Care Coordinators
Documentation

The care coordination team should use standard documentation templates whenever possible and document within the same system. As mentioned earlier, the three basic templates are for post-acute care/emergency room visits, post-subacute/rehabilitation records, and high-risk patient care.

The care coordination team should use templates for all calls and in-person meetings with patients. Using documentation tools with designated cells allows data to be pulled and used to help to guide future care. For example, if there is a question on the template that prompts the care coordinator to ask a patient after hospitalization, "Do you understand how and when to take your medications?" Then your organization can evaluate how well the patients are being educated on medication usage before leaving the hospital.

Standardization of templates is also a great way to teach new care coordinators what is important when communicating with patients. Of course, there should always be space to allow the care coordinator to elaborate with free text.

Resources and Directories

In order for a care coordinator to function and assist patients, several resource guides will be required. These should be given to the staff in electronic and paper format. The basic guides that are required are the following:

- Community resources: everything from durable medical equipment referrals, transportation, and food services to financial assistance
- Internal organization resources: IT assistance, HR, and supervisor contacts, for example
- Provider/practice information for the entire organization: to help when covering days off/vacation or changes in assignment
- Post-acute contact information: rehabilitation centers, nursing homes, SNFs, and visiting nursing services, for example

The care coordinators will use resources and contact information each day. It is important that the guides are updated at least every six months, if not quarterly. This is mostly due to staff turnover in the post-acute settings.

Quality Metrics: Care Coordinator Responsibilities

Every organization is following some type of quality metric requirement. The care coordinator can assist their practices in collecting and documenting the metrics correctly, although it should not be the main responsibility of the coordinator. The practices should "own" metric collection in order to perform at high levels on a consistent basis. If metric collection is left to one or two people, what happens when those people have vacation or terminate employment completely?

The care coordinator should work with the providers and staff within the practice to ensure a workflow is established and executed for each metric. In my organization, each year we create what we call a "Collaborative Workflow Agreement for Quality Metrics." The care coordination team works with the practice to establish exactly how each metric will be collected (i.e., at what time, by whom, where it is documented), and it is written in the agreement and signed by the providers and staff. Each month a random sample of patients is audited for these metrics and the results (with provider and staff names) are shared with all. This ensures that each month the practice leadership and staff are aware of metric performance and can refer back to the collaborative agreement to see where the process of metric collection broke down if the audit is poor. This monthly audit is also sent to ACO leadership by each practice and aggregated as a whole so that there are no surprise poor performers in the yearly metric audit or group practice reporting option (used to report quality metric results to Medicare).

In my organization, we have created a secondary embedded practice role called a transition assistant (TA) who takes more responsibility for assisting the practice to document quality metrics and is the primary source for mining the metrics when needed and transferring the data to the correct person/payer. This position is best for a medical assistant–type full-time equivalent who has worked in a physician practice and is comfortable with medical terminology and office workflows. The TA is the one who actually performs the monthly open chart audit for the practice and completes what we call a "Huddle List." The Huddle List is completed for patients with appointments for the following day. The patient schedule notes the quality metrics that should be documented or collected during the visit. In most practices, the medical assisting staff, RN staff, and doctors receive a copy of this and use their established workflows within the collaborative agreement to ensure the metrics are collected and documented correctly.

We have also requested that each practice designate an "ACO champion." This is a point person who the practice believes is in the best position to assist the care coordinator in creating and enforcing work-flows that support value-based care as well as population management principles. This person should exert a positive influence over the practice staff and setting and also answer questions on ACO metrics and work-flows when the care coordinator or transition assistant are not present.

Monitoring Care Coordinator Productivity and Activities

Monitoring productivity is a challenge in care coordination. When the care coordinators are embedded in community practices, it is even more challenging because you are not directly observing your staff. Some patients will require multiple calls and outreaches while others will not, so a simple count of calls made or notes written will not give a complete assessment of a care coordinators productivity or impact on a population of patients.

Also, outcome data cannot be solely relied upon due to noncompli-ance instances of the patient, provider, or practice. Noncompliance can alter length-of-stay measurement, clinical quality metrics, and financial metrics.

There is no "right" number for measuring productivity, although the number of contacts the care coordinator is making should be measur-able by the documentation system used, which is an objective measure-ment of overall productivity. The following is what I use in my orga-nization as evidence of highly effective care coordination:

1. All calls and attempted calls to patients, providers, and services are documented within Healthy Planet, a part of our electronic health record.
2. At all times the care coordinator has an updated list of all patients in transition from the hospital to home. It is available to share with management and ACO providers at any time.
3. They have the ability to contact and track patients through transitions from hospital to home by using multiple modalities of ADT sources to accommodate the population served in the assigned ACO practices.

4. The number of phone calls/outreaches to patients is meeting expectations.
5. The number of care plans created and updated is meeting expectations.
6. High-risk patient responsibilities are completed.
7. Quality of notes is established in a review of documentation on a regular basis.

ACO management will also review individual care coordinator performance with assigned practices and service/vendor colleagues. Performance standards will be based on expectations as well as customer service elements. The customer is defined as the practice staff, physicians, and patients.

Care Coordinator Expectations

The most effective way I have found to relay and hold care coordination staff accountable is to have regular meetings with an agenda and meeting minutes. When starting a meeting program, run them weekly in the beginning, then taper to biweekly, and finally to monthly. Discussion in the meeting should offer the staff more time to speak than the leader. You will create the best workflows and policies if you give your staff the goal and allow them to contribute on how to reach it. They are the ones doing the work each day. They will eventually teach you more than any article, conference, course, or so-called expert. They know their practices, the organization, and the barriers better than anyone. Listen to your staff.

It is also important to meet with staff individually in their practice setting in order to completely understand the challenges your staff face. For example, our organization is in its sixth year, and I still have staff that are not given space in practices. They move with cell phones and laptops from the practice kitchen to exam rooms to waiting rooms throughout the day at the practice's discretion. Obviously, I can't expect this staff to accomplish as much as the care coordinators who have their own desk, chair, desktop computer with two screens, and landline telephone.

Working with Practices

To begin embedded care coordination on a positive note, it is best for the organization management to meet with the practice physicians and staff *before* the care coordinator arrives for his or her first day of work. Staff buy-in to the ACO and to the coordinator's role is essential for the program to be effective. The practice staff and providers must understand exactly what the care coordinator's role is and how they are directly taking care of patients or assisting the practice to improve patient care—both on individual patients and on the entire practice panel.

Here are some suggestions on how to embed care coordinators:

1. Start with practices that are open to the concept of care coordination within their offices and have the space to accommodate a coordinator. This would include, at minimum, a chair and a desk or other dedicated work space in an area where they have access to the clinical staff. Once you have success in this type of office, you can use these practices as references for other offices that are hesitant to have an embedded care coordinator.

2. The care coordinator should shadow the entire practice staff for at least one to two hours. This gives the coordinators a chance to personally meet the staff and understand how their role fits into the overall workflow of the practice. At the same time, it gives the care coordinator the opportunity to explain his or her role and answer any questions. Most importantly, it gives the care coordinator a chance to make acquaintances and develop an early working relationship. The key to successful embedment is for the care coordinator to become part of the *practice culture*. This approach is a solid step toward care coordination acceptance.

3. ACO management should check in with practice management after the first day, at the end of the first week, and then weekly for a month. Although you may think the practice had a good understanding of the care coordinator's role and responsibilities, there are always misunderstandings. If there is not clarification

early, this can lead to confusion, resentment, and even anger, which will be taken out directly on the care coordinator.

4. Work with the care coordinator to demonstrate his or her worth as soon as possible. The practices must be taught and then frequently reminded that care coordination is there as a resource for them. They should use the coordinator for communication with and tracking of patients in transition from hospital to home as well as for those patients who are complex and need more clinical and social management than the traditional office staff can support.

....

The following pages come from an internal document created to explain the care coordinator theory of my current organization as well as a few of the workflows that support the theory. The workflows have resulted in successful shared savings with each year of participation in the Medicare Shared Savings Program.

Care Coordination: Implementation and Assessment

Care coordination in the Hackensack Meridian outpatient practice environment is a comprehensive program focused on delivering high-value care. Since 2012, the Hackensack ACO has successfully improved clinical outcomes of individuals and communities, improved patient experience, and decreased the total cost of care by creating effective and efficient care delivery systems. Early adoption of value-based care principles and a desire to be a national leader in the transformation of health care has made the Hackensack Alliance ACO one of the most successful ACO organizations in the country. Coordinating care has been a significant factor in our success and will become more important as the ACO continues to grow.

This manual contains key components to understanding the role and function of a care coordinator within the ACO. Additionally, there will be both formal and informal training to ensure each care coordinator understands the responsibilities and outcome measures expected from this role.

$$\text{High Value Care} = \frac{\text{Quality of Care}}{\text{Cost of Care}}$$

To deliver high value health care, the care coordination team must focus on increasing the quality of care provided while keeping costs controlled.

Care Coordination Role and Responsibilities

As a Hackensack Meridian care coordinator, you will be responsible for a group of patients with diverse social and medical issues. The scope and depth of services delivered will be dependent on the patient. Many patients only need yearly physicals and preventative services while other patients will require more time and services. A good example of this is patients who are transitioning from hospital to home. Then there are those patients with multiple chronic conditions, which will require even more care coordination support to ensure that providers are speaking to each other, social services are in place, and family and caregivers (if involved) are also educated and supported.

A care coordinator's main objective will be to ensure that each patient is receiving appropriate services that optimize their current health status.

In order to consistently deliver high value and quality care, the patient's needs and preferences must be known to all those providing care. This requires the right people, at the right time, having information to guide high-quality, appropriate care. The care coordinator is one of the most important members of the ACO team to ensure this communication occurs. In an ACO, the primary care provider (PCP) is designated as the provider who coordinates all medical care for each patient. Your main objective is to assist the PCP to successfully do this by supporting the transmission of pertinent patient information between providers so that patients may receive high-quality, efficient care. Multiple workflows, software, templates, and tools have been created to assist the care coordinator and these tools will be introduced upon orientation to the ACO. The role of the care coordinator can be further understood by reviewing the general overarching responsibilities and utilizing the standardized workflows created to support the most common patient types and situations you will be managing.

Overarching Responsibilities of the Care Coordinator

- Engaging the patient in the development of an individualized care plan that reflects his or her health care needs and priorities
- Educating patients and caregivers on preventative services as well as disease process and management as indicated
- Ensuring that patients understand their roles outlined in their care plans and feel equipped to fulfill their responsibilities
- Identifying all of the barriers—psychological, social, financial, and environmental—that affect the patient's ability to adhere to treatments or maintain their health
- Assisting the primary care physician in assembling the appropriate team of health care professionals to address a patient's needs
- Facilitating appropriate and timely communication between care team members
- Assisting the primary care physician with optimizing site of care for patient needs
- Following up with patients periodically to ensure their needs are being met and that their circumstances and priorities have not changed
- Oversight of the transitional assistant(s) assigned to your practices in regard to metric gap completion

Care Coordination Functions Support the Overall Goals of the ACO

All of a care coordinator's interactions with patients and practices should support the ACOs goals and guiding principles listed below:

- Reduction in overall cost of care
- Reductions in hospital admissions and emergency room visits
- Improved overall quality of care
- Increased patient-perceived experience/satisfaction
- Decreases in medication costs
- Increased patient confidence in managing self-care

Care Coordination Workflows

Although it is not possible to document a specific procedure for every patient situation you will encounter, there are established standardized workflows that the care coordinator should utilize that cover much of a typical workday.

The following are examples of established workflows.

Patients Admitted to an Acute Care Facility

1. Review admitted patients to any acute care facility daily where ACO has access.
2. Review patient's admitting diagnosis, plan of care, and any discharge needs at that time.
3. Consider contacting the patient's family member or patient themselves to discuss current concerns, communication with PCP, and discharge needs.
4. Reach out to inpatient case manager/social worker to offer information on past medical care. Specifically review the following:
   a. Discharge plan: confirm appropriateness
   b. Appointments with PCP and specialists post-discharge
   c. Out-of-bed order/physical therapy evaluation if not contraindicated
5. If patient is being considered for subacute facility, confirm that this is an appropriate step for their discharge needs.
6. If able, visit patient in hospital.

Patient's Post–Emergency Room Visit

1. Review ADT system(s) and reports for patients seen in the emergency room.
2. Call patients post-ER as soon as possible but no more than five business days to follow up on:
   a. Indication for visit
   b. Follow-up on outstanding care issues
   c. Ensure patient has follow-up visit with provider
3. If ER visit does not seem appropriate, educate patient on contacting the provider and addressing symptoms early rather than waiting until there is no other alternative than to go to ER.
4. Document call and ensure provider has a copy of documentation in practice's electronic medical record.
5. Two call attempts on consecutive days should be placed to the patient. If the patient does not answer, work with the office staff to continue to complete a successful call.

Patient Admitted to a Subacute Care Facility

1. The Care Coordination Hand-off Tool should be completed and sent to the receiving facility within 24 hours of discharge from the acute care setting.
2. Once patient has been transferred, direct contact should occur between the care coordinator and the designated employee(s) at the facility to review plan of care, support at home, and any discharge needs. Consider communication to director of nursing for any medical or nursing needs.
3. Social worker is to be urged to arrange a family meeting within the first 72 hours of patient's arrival; this family meeting should take place within the first five business days of patient's admission to the facility.
4. Estimated date of transition home should be established during family meeting and for all disciplines involved in order to anticipate an appropriate length of stay.

5. Care coordinator should have a minimum of weekly communication with all disciplines in subacute facilities.
6. The care coordinator will conduct a combination of the below activities while patient is in SNF care:
   a. Be an active participant in the family meeting if time allows.
   b. Reinforce expectation of facility to notify care coordinator if patient's status or discharge date/plan changes.
7. Care coordinator to communicate with patient and patient's family members and establish relationship to confirm smooth transition home or into long-term care facility.

Patient Transitioned Home

1. Once patient has transitioned back to their home setting, the first follow-up call should occur within the first 24 hours and no later than 48 hours. This follow-up call should include the following:
   a. Utilize the discharge call template for the first call. Continue to utilize this template if the patient is high risk.
   b. Perform medication reconciliation. Review with patient and/or caregiver medication name, dose, reason for medication, schedule of medications, and possible side effects of each medication. Use teach-back approach.
   c. Make appointment for follow-up visit with ACO physician within one week.
   d. Collaborate with provider for any concerns to address in a timely manner.
   e. Assist patient with making follow-up appointments with specialists currently involved in the care of the patient.
   f. Assess newly discovered discharge needs.
   g. Arrange for any additional needs or durable medical equipment at home.
   h. Review signs and symptoms of chronic condition and/or what originally brought them to the hospital. Provide education for symptom recognition and self-care instructions.

    i. Review when appropriate to utilize emergency services vs. primary care physician office.

2. Evaluate if/when follow-up call should be made to patient and/or caregiver. Document plan for calls.

3. Whenever possible, meet with patient and caregiver face-to-face during the follow-up visit for clarification of plan of care, medication review, and to answer any questions or concerns.

Patients with Visiting Nurse Services

1. Establish communication with primary nurse within the visiting nurse service. Review plan of care, estimated length of stay, and any needs the patient may have at home.

2. Communicate the expectation of notification when changes in plan of care occur or when new issues arrive.

3. Remain in contact with the patient throughout visiting nursing services.

4. Remind visiting nursing services to notify ACO upon last visit.

5. Contact patient and make an appointment for ACO physician within one week.

High-Risk Patient Management

1. Patients will be contacted a minimum of once quarterly.
   a. Contacts can be from the ACO staff, practice staff, an ACO physician, or an office visit, but the care coordinator must verify there was contact and the patient is not having issues or complications.
   b. The standardized high-risk note will be utilized for outreach calls to patients (see figure 3.1).

2. A care plan is completed and updated a minimum of once quarterly.

3. An annual wellness visit is completed each year.

4. High-risk patients upon discharge from the hospital, rehabilitation facility, or skilled nursing facility are followed up by the care

Time taken: 0902   ⊘   4/26/2017 📅   Show: ☐ Row Info ☐ Last Filed ☐ Details ☑ All Choices

☻ Values By   ✚ Create Note

High-Risk Call	To be used by the care coordinator for all high-risk patients All questions are required
How have you been doing since the last time we spoke?	☐ N/A – first time speaking with patient/caregiver
	Patient has specific complaints – see below for details
	Patient/caregiver states that overall doing well – no significant complaints

Recent hospitalizations/ER visits	Ask if there were any hospital or ER visits since the last time you spoke to patient or since last time patient was in the office.
	☐ Patient states no ER or hospital admissions
	Patient states ER and/or hospital visit – see below for details
	Include place, date, and reason for ER/hospital

Specialist, diagnostics, or other appointments attended recently or scheduled	☐ None
	Yes – see text below

Future appointments	
Ensure patient has a follow-up appointment with physician(s) scheduled and is able to attend	☐ Yes, has appointment and transportation to office/clinic
	Yes, patient has appointment but no transportation – see text below
	No, patient does not have appointment – see text below
	Patient/caregiver refused to discuss
	No PCP visit in 3 months – appointment made
	No PCP visit in 3 months – appointment not made – see text below
	Other – see text

Medication verification/changes	
Review that patient has obtained and is taking all medications as ordered	☐ Yes, taking medications correctly – no changes
	Yes, has medications but may not be taking correctly – education given
	No, patient does not have meds or is not taking meds – see text below
	Medications have been changed – see text

Support System	
Ensure patient has support at home	☐ Caregiver in home with patient
	Caregiver lives close
	No caregiver support
	Other – see text

Figure 3.1. Documentation template for high-risk patient calls.

⊞ Hackensack ACO High-Risk Call Template

Time taken: 0902 ⊘ 4/26/2017 📅   Show: ☐ Row Info   ☐ Last Filed   ☐ Details   ☑ All Choices

⧎ Values By   ✚ Create Note

Activities of daily living (ADLs)

Inquire as to ability to perform activities of daily living

🗋
Patient is able to perform ADLs independently
Patient has assistance performing ADLs
Patient is having difficulty with ADLs – no assistance currently available – see text
Other – see text

Is visiting nursing service or home health ordered?

🗋
Yes
No

Necessary equipment/services

Ensure patient has been prescribed necessary medical/functional equipment and services. Check off if patient is currently in need(s) of the following and plan to assist patient with the need(s)

🗋
Prescribed medical equipment — specify below
Transportation
Medication retrieval
Groceries/food
Safe housing
Other – see text
Patient has no equipment or service needs at this time

Patient concerns related to health

Ask of expectations and goals and how you can assist

🗋
Patient/caregiver has no concerns
Patient/caregiver stated concerns – see text

Symptom recognition

Based on current issue(s) and medical history – patient is aware of symptoms to report to MD

Based on current issue(s) and medical history – patient is aware of symptoms to report to MD

🗋
Patient/caregiver is aware of symptoms to report to MD
Patient/caregiver is not aware of symptoms to report to MD – patient educated – see text below
Patient/caregiver currently having symptoms and MD to be notified – see text below
Other – see text

Follow-up and plan for patient:

Create/update or add care plan(s) on each contact

Figure 3.1. *(continued)*

coordinator via telephone, and the patient has an office visit within three to seven days of discharge. Fourteen days maximum to comply with transitional coding and ensure timely follow-up. If patient refuses office visit—this is documented.

5. Quality metrics are up to date.
    a. Must work with practice to ensure compliance. If a metric is not met, there is documentation of reason.
    b. This is a transition assistant task, but the care coordinator has ultimate responsibility.
6. Applicable community resources are offered to patients.
7. When possible, care coordinator to meet with patient during the office visit.

Population Health Management Responsibilities

Most of the tasks in population health are completed by the transition assistant and are outlined below. However, it is the care coordinators responsibility to oversee that the transition assistant is completing metrics. If there is a deficit in metrics, this is to be reported to ACO management immediately.

1. Obtain list of attributed patients from each insurance payer.
2. Assist practice in developing a workflow to ensure all patients are "touched" by the practice.
    a. Assist practice to schedule and complete a yearly physical for each patient
    b. Ensure a workflow is created for each individual quality measure, and use a Collaborative Workflow Agreement.
3. Perform the monthly audit of clinical records for gaps in quality care measures. This will be shared with ACO management and leadership as well as the individual practice.
4. Create a corrective plan with the practice to facilitate collections of required quality metrics.
5. Contact ACO patients to make appointments for outstanding preventative care measures and annual physical appointments.

6. Compile list of patients with missing measures and develop a plan to reduce the numerator.

Chronic-Stable Patient Management Responsibilities

1. Patients with chronic conditions who are stable, in that there are no signs symptoms or diagnostics of disease progression, should have two yearly visits minimum with the ACO primary care provider (PCP).
2. These visits should be completed even if a specialist is managing most of the patient's care. It is important that the PCP is kept informed of patient status and that preventative services and screenings continue to be completed.
3. All consults and office notes of specialists should be retrieved and placed in the patient's chart. The care coordinator should work with the office staff and the transition assistant to ensure there is a workflow to support this.

Interactions and Communication with Key ACO Staff and Physicians

A care coordinator's success within a practice is highly dependent on how well he or she communicates and develops good working relationships with the ACO practice. The coordinator will be in daily communication with physicians and ACO practice staff in order to coordinate services and care. There will also be an ongoing responsibility for workflow training, monitoring and providing feedback on how the practice is performing on ACO quality metrics, and educating practice staff on ACO standards (figure 3.2).

Monitor and Provide Feedback to Physicians and Practice Staff

It will be necessary for the care coordinator to adjust ACO concepts to the level of his or her audience. All staff and physicians will require a

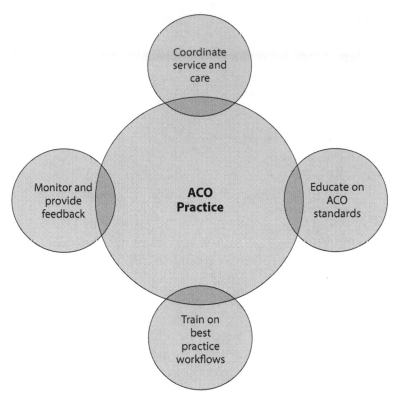

Figure 3.2. Essential communication responsibilities of the care coordinator in an accountable care organization (ACO) practice.

strong understanding as to the purpose and goals of the ACO as well as understanding the specific functions of the care coordinators within their practice.

Upon first working with either an existing ACO practice or a new ACO practice, it is important for the care coordinator to shadow all positions, from the front desk staff to the physicians. This is the best way to understand how the office functions. The care coordinator can then provide added benefit of the practice. You, the care coordinator, also should use this time to communicate and gain feedback as to how to best work with each area within the practice.

Individualize Practice Workflows

ACO interventions and workflows that support ACO goals must be individualized to fit the needs of each practice. Although standardization is important, some level of individualism must occur for practices to experience a fluid adjustment into the ACO.

A good example of this concept is how staffing can impact ACO workflows. Some practices have a full complement of staff, including front desk, billers, managers, nurses, medical assistants, nurse practitioners, and physicians. Other practice locations may have only a front desk person, a medical assistant, and a physician who each function in various roles to complete what the manager, nurse, and billers do in other practice locations. The care coordinator must assist the minimally staffed practice to develop a variation of workflow that will still support ACO practice requirements.

Practice Engagement Concepts

Care coordinators are placed into practices with diverse levels of exposure to the value-based care principles that are foundational to ACOs. This may result in the care coordinator experiencing different levels of engagement between practices and even different levels of engagement within the same individual practice.

When you encounter resistance, it is best to continue to gently remind the staff of the indications for required workflows and information. If this is not effective, notify the care coordination management to engage with the practice. Change is sometimes difficult, especially when current practices have been used for many years.

....

Key Concepts for Successful Care Coordination
Use a Care Coordination Model that Truly Suits Your Organization

Designing a care coordination model that suits your unique organization may require that you do not replicate published models exactly but instead modify them to fit the circumstances of your patient population and care sites. Be sure there are standardized and measurable interventions that can be tracked and assessed for impact on your population's overall health status. For example, you implemented a workflow that every patient should be called post–ER visits and then followed up. After a period of six months or one year, have ER visits decreased? If not, consider reviewing the workflow. Should you alter or eliminate this intervention? Every intervention you use should have a measurable goal tied to it.

Build and Maintain Relationships with Care Continuum Partners on All Levels

It is important to have good relations and communications with your care partners at every level from executive to frontline staff. Take time whenever possible to have face-to-face meetings and review what is and is not working. Then, how can you work *together* to improve the workflows? This will lead to increased patient satisfaction and also promote improved staff and provider experiences

Provide forums where frontline staff from separate organizations can meet—for example, the ACO care coordinators and the nurses from the home care agency, or the ACO care coordinators and the inpatient case management nurses from a hospital. They can meet together with or without executive management oversight. Such a meeting will lead to stronger relationship building that knocks down the "us versus them" concept, which is so frequently seen in health care.

At the executive level, it will always be necessary to check in to be sure that your partners remain satisfied with the collaborative arrangements and that your incentives remain aligned.

Provide the Right Tools for the Care Coordination Team to Get the Job Done

Spend time choosing software and computer equipment that will truly assist the care coordinators to manage patients. The difference between what vendors claim to deliver and what they actually do deliver is remarkable. Insist on speaking to and visiting other ACOs who utilize the vendor's products. Be sure, above all else, that the care coordinators evaluate all potential software/computer equipment and that their opinions on purchase are heavily weighted.

Empower, Trust, and Support Your Team

Much of my early success was due to the fact that I was given the autonomy to hire who I believed would do the best job, create the initial workflows that I believed would serve us best, and work with vendors that I believed would truly support our organization. I was empowered and supported by this volume's editor, Dr. Peter Gross. He believed in me and trusted my instincts, which led to the great success of our care coordination program.

I have carried on this leadership style with my own staff. When there is a problem to be solved, a new goal to be met, or anything new that will directly affect the care coordinator's job, I rely heavily on their insight and input to assist with how to move forward. It has been shown that when employees are involved in making decisions, they then feel commitment to the overall success of the organization. This leads to increased productivity because they want to see their ideas succeed. This also benefits overall morale, increased job satisfaction, and prepares your team for additional responsibility in the future (5, 6).

REFERENCES
1. Berkowitz SA, Parashuram S, Rowan K, et al. Association of a care coordination model with health care costs and utilization: the Johns Hopkins Community Health Partnership (J-CHiP). *JAMA Netw Open.* 2018;1(7):e184273. doi:10.1001/jamanetworkopen.2018.4273.
2. Rundall TG, Wu FM, Lewis VA, Schoenherr KE, Shortell SM. Contributions of relational coordination to care management in accountable care organizations: views of managerial and clinical leaders. *Health Care Manage Rev.* 2016;41(2):88–100. doi:10.1097/HMR.0000000000000064.
3. Huber TP, Shortell SM, Rodriguez HP. Improving care transitions management: examining the role of accountable care organization participation and expanded electronic health record functionality. *Health Serv Res.* 2017;52(4):1494–1510. doi:10.1111/1475-6773.12546.

4. Kripalani S, Theobald CN, Anctil B, Vasilevskis EE. Reducing hospital readmission rates: current strategies and future directions. *Annu Rev Med.* 2014;65:471–485. doi:10.1146/annurev-med-022613-090415.

5. Juneja P. Advantages and disadvantages of participative management. Management Study Guide website. https://www.managementstudyguide.com /participative-management-advantages-disadvantages.htm. Accessed February 15, 2019.

6. Anderson C. The advantages of employee involvement in decision making. *Small Business Chron.* March 4, 2019. https://smallbusiness.chron.com/advantages -employee-involvement-decision-making-18264.html. Accessed February 15, 2019.

FOUR

Quality Measurement in Accountable Care Organizations

GUY D'ANDREA AND KRIS CORWIN

*Guy has worked with numerous public and private health quality
organizations and is well versed in how quality measures are created and
implemented for accountable care organizations (ACOs). Prioritizing
compliance with the Centers for Medicare and Medicaid Services (CMS)
quality measure set will pave the way to your success as an ACO.*

Introduction

Quality measurement is fundamental to the concept of ACOs. Indeed,
the term *accountable* care organization raises the question, "Accountable for what?" The short answer is "quality and cost." In fact, these
two goals are highly linked. Many quality measures, such as avoidance
of unplanned hospitalizations for patients with chronic diseases, generate costs savings as a by-product. It is this connection between quality
and cost that defines expectations for ACOs.

The high cost of health care is a well-known fact. Anyone who pays for
health insurance understands that health care is very expensive and that
the cost is rising. As of 2017, the United States spends over $10,000 per
capita on health care, among the most when comparing industrialized nations (1). Less well known is that the quality of health care in the United
States often lags other countries, especially for long-term management of
complex patients, such as the chronically ill. Together, the combination of
low quality and high cost means that employers, patients, and taxpayers
are getting poor value for their health care spending. ACOs are intended
to change that, and quality measures are central to that mission.

The first step to improving performance is to define and measure it.
An ACO can measure whether patients get the right diagnostic tests or

the right services and support to manage their health needs. An ACO can measure avoidance of unnecessary health services that add cost without improving care. Alternatively, an ACO can measure whether patients are achieving good outcomes. Selecting good measures lets doctors and hospitals know what they are expected to do and provides a mechanism to track how well they do it.

The next step for an ACO is to connect measures to programs that motivate performance. In some cases, external accountability programs, such as Medicare, private health plans, or large employers, will require specific measures. Many ACOs adjust payments to doctors and hospitals based on their performance. In other cases, you might use measures for internal tracking and quality improvement efforts. The measure sets for these various purposes may overlap but do not need to be identical. In selecting a set of measures to collect, track, and report, you need to balance the expectations of external stakeholders and the imperatives in internal management. Administrative feasibility is also a factor, as physicians have limited bandwidth to report data or interpret results. To select the right measures, you need to understand the role and use of quality measures, and the measures that apply to their patient populations.

Focus on Quality Measures

In the mid-1990s, few Americans would have disagreed with the statement, "The United States has the best quality of care in the world." While the cost of care was a problem then (as it is still), gaps in the quality of care were not well recognized. This began to change in 1999, with the publication of the landmark report *To Err Is Human: Building a Safer Health System* by the Institute of Medicine (IOM). The report documented the significant harm done to patients from medical errors and launched some of the early national efforts to measure and publicly report the performance of health care providers. For example, large employers founded the Leapfrog Group in 2000 to collect measures of hospital safety.

In 2001, the IOM released a follow-up report, *Crossing the Quality Chasm: A New Health System for the 21st Century*. This report expanded on the IOM's previous work and documented more pervasive gaps in health care delivery across the care continuum. *Crossing the Quality Chasm* described the ways in which the US health care system failed to meet the needs of patients, especially those with complex and ongoing health care needs (2). These findings were reinforced in 2003 with the publication of "The Quality of Health Care Delivered to Adults in the United States" in the *New England Journal of Medicine*. This study found that patients received recommended, evidence-based care only about half of the time. Quality varied substantially across different medical conditions. In summary, the study found that "deficits . . . in adherence to recommended processes for basic care pose serious threats to the health of the American public" (3).

In the years since these landmark reports, researchers have continued to study and track quality of care. For example, in its *Why Not the Best?* reports (4), the Commonwealth Fund tracks US health system performance on key indicators compared to other developed countries. In addition, the Kaiser Family Foundation issues frequent reports on quality topics that cite ongoing deficits in health care quality (5). While these studies show that there are still significant gaps in quality for many patients, newer studies also show that the health system is making progress on many key quality indicators. A 2018 CMS report (6) found the following effects estimated from improved national rates for key indicators:

- 670,000 additional patients with controlled blood pressure (2006–2015)
- 510,000 fewer patients with poor diabetes control (2006–2015)
- 12,000 fewer deaths following hospitalization for a heart attack (2008–2015)
- 70,000 fewer unplanned readmissions (2011–2015)
- 840,000 fewer pressure ulcers among nursing home residents (2011–2015)
- Nearly nine million more hospitalized patients with a highly favorable experience with their hospital (2008–2015)

Oversight of Quality Measures

In the 1990s, as growing evidence pointed to quality gaps in health care, key stakeholder groups identified that measurement was critical to driving quality improvement. Therefore, infrastructure and processes were necessary to oversee the development and dissemination of measures. The purposes of such an infrastructure would be to ensure that measures met criteria for scientific validity and promote consistency in measurement across different providers and care settings.

A key step in developing the necessary infrastructure was the formation of the National Quality Forum (NQF). The NQF was created in 1999 by a coalition of public- and private-sector leaders. The coalition was called the President's Advisory Commission on Consumer Protection and Quality in the Health Care Industry. It concluded that an organization was needed to promote and ensure patient protections and health care quality through measurement and public reporting (7). The federal government and many other entities now rely on NQF-endorsed measures as evidence-based approaches to improving care. Today, about 300 NQF-endorsed measures are used in more than 20 federal public reporting and pay-for-performance programs as well as in private-sector and state programs. Additionally, the Department of Health and Human Services relies on the guidance of NQF's Measure Applications Partnership to foster the use of a more uniform set of measures across federal programs that provide health coverage for about 120 million Americans.

Measures are conceived, developed, tested, and maintained by a wide range of health organizations. These include physician specialty societies, nonprofit organizations, government agencies, hospitals and physician groups, accreditation bodies, and others. Typically, these organizations develop measures relevant to their area of focus. For example, the American Society of Clinical Oncology has developed numerous measures for cancer treatment. The American Heart Association has developed measures for cardiovascular care. More recently, the International Consortium for Health Outcomes Measurement has promoted the adoption of measure sets focused on patient outcomes. The list of measure developers is extensive and constantly evolving as various organizations seek to fill gaps in measurement and advance measurement science.

Regardless of their origin, many measures intended for use in public reporting or accountability programs are submitted to the NQF for review. The NQF criteria address factors such as the scientific validity of a measure, feasibility for implementation, and importance to patient outcomes. Measures that meet the criteria receive NQF endorsement. As of early 2018, the NQF had endorsed over 700 measures, covering a broad range of health care topics such as chronic care management, inpatient care, and care coordination. New measures are continually being developed, endorsed, and implemented (8).

Measure Sets

When measures are put into use, they are typically assembled into measure sets that span the different services and outcomes a health care provider is expected to achieve. For example, a measure set for diabetes care might include measures for blood pressure screening and control, blood sugar screening and control, smoking cessation, and monitoring for complications. A provider subject to the measure set would be evaluated on each individual measure, and then the measure results would be aggregated into an overall score. (There are numerous different methods for combining measure results into an aggregate score. Such methods are outside the scope of this chapter.) The overall score might be reported to patients, or it could be used to determine eligibility for financial incentives.

Measure sets are especially important for ACOs, given the broad range of populations and health care services that ACOs must manage. Most ACO measure sets include measures of primary care access, chronic care management, preventable health utilization, overall cost, and patient satisfaction. Given the long list of potential measures, one of your biggest challenges is to build a measure set broad enough for your ACO's whole population yet short enough to be administratively feasible.

For the various Medicare ACO programs, CMS determines the measure set. For private-sector ACO programs, the measure set is negotiated between your ACO and the health plan. The measure set is frequently based on the Medicare model. Notably, the Medicare ACO measure sets do not include maternity care or pediatric measures, so you should consider these for inclusion if appropriate to the population. Table 4.1 shows the most current measure set in use for Medicare ACOs.

Table 4.1. Accountable care organization measures used in the Medicare Shared Savings Program for 2019

Domain	Measure ID	Measure name
Patient/caregiver experience (using survey data collected from patients by the Centers for Medicare and Medicaid)	ACO 1	Getting timely care, appointments, and information
	ACO 2	How well your providers communicate
	ACO 3	Patients' rating of provider
	ACO 4	Access to specialists
	ACO 5	Health promotion and education
	ACO 6	Shared decision-making
	ACO 7	Health status and functional status
	ACO 34	Stewardship of patient resources
	ACO 45	Courteous and helpful office staff
	ACO 46	Care coordination
Care coordination and patient safety	ACO 8	Risk standardized, all condition readmissions
	ACO 38	All-cause unplanned admissions for patients with multiple chronic conditions
	ACO 43	Ambulatory sensitive condition acute composite
	ACO 13	Falls: screening for future fall risk
Preventive health	ACO 14	Preventive care and screening: influenza immunization
	ACO 17	Preventive care and screening: tobacco use screening and cessation intervention
	ACO 18	Preventive care and screening: screening for clinical depression and follow-up plan
	ACO 19	Colorectal cancer screening
	ACO 20	Breast cancer screening
	ACO 42	Statin therapy for the prevention and treatment of cardiovascular disease
At-risk population: depression	ACO 40	Depression remission at 12 months
At-risk population: diabetes	ACO 27	Diabetes mellitus: hemoglobin A1c poor control
At-risk population: hypertension	ACO 28	Hypertension: controlling high blood pressure

Source: Centers for Medicare and Medicaid Services (CMS). *Medicare Shared Savings Program, Quality Measurement Methodology and Resources: Specifications Applicable for Performance Year 2019.* Baltimore, MD: CMS; May 2019. https://www.cms.gov/Medicare/Medicare-Fee-for-Service-Payment /sharedsavingsprogram/Downloads/quality-measurement-methodology-and-resources.pdf. Accessed October 23, 2019.

Note: CMS has removed or replaced certain measures since first implementing the ACO measure sets, so the list has a nonsequential numbering order. CMS updates the list of ACO measures annually, adding new measures, updating existing measures, and retiring some measures. Please refer to the CMS website (www.cms.gov) for the latest information.

Quality Improvement Process

In addition to supporting external accountability, quality measures also support internal improvement efforts. "Plan-Do-Study-Act" is a widely accepted approach to continuous quality improvement (9). Some form of this cycle takes place within all ACOs. A quality improvement plan for an ACO will have as its chief goal to boost performance on the measure set it has negotiated with payers/purchasers. Once in a defined risk-sharing arrangement, you must organize and improve care using the results of measurement as the keys to monitoring organizational effectiveness. Because measure sets used in arrangements with payers and providers are agreed upon to reasonably share risk for improving the health of the ACO population, measurement results can provide insight on actual and expected financial performance. You might prioritize resources for quality improvement activities based on areas that create the most risk (financial loss) or provide the best opportunity to share in savings (financial gain). ACO leaders ask where the gaps in quality performance exist and then explore how to close those gaps. Performing a gap analysis will help you triage internal quality improvement needs. You can base an action plan on these priorities as a foundation for selecting the right interventions.

Accountability Measures

Internal quality improvement needs arise under every setting and every level of care included in the ACO entity. You can best meet these needs with indicators and tools for measurement that are important for assessing processes and structure that lead to better outcomes. These internal improvement measures may have results that can be rolled up into accountability measures or support performance on accountability measures, but they are not typically reported to the payers or public. Internal quality measurement is about monitoring progress toward goals that ACO leaders have set for the organization.

Using performance on the accountability measures in the ACO measure sets, you can identify corresponding measurement opportunities for internal accountability measures. These measures will directly contribute to boosting your external measures while monitoring progress toward quality improvement across the organization. Within the organization, quality improvement teams conduct continuous process improvement cycles, planning and studying what internal quality efforts are expected to improve internal accountability measures.

For example, your ACO may identify that it needs to improve care delivered to patients with diabetes. An internal quality improvement team engaged in continuous quality improvement plans a project to test if patients with diabetes have adequate monitoring—such as routine visits and blood work. The improvement activity results in data showing a certain subset of the diabetic population within your ACO frequently misses appointments and has significantly poorer control of their blood glucose levels. Your ACO would then focus a quality improvement initiative to coordinate appointments and ensure blood work is done regularly. The quality improvement team refines interventions.

Using the same hypothetical, if missed appointments come down but the better results do not lead to improvement on accountability measures, then your team can examine other areas. Such additional efforts could mean more comprehensive, interdisciplinary care through group visits and community partners to both increase reach and minimize costs. The preceding example also illustrates that internal improvement may not immediately generate positive results, so your ACO must be willing to accept risk and remain flexible in its approach to quality improvement.

Keys to Success

Quality measurement and improvement is a central pillar of the ACO model. Government purchasers and commercial insurers expect ACOs to improve care delivery and coordination in order to drive better population outcomes. Defining and understanding relevant quality measures is the first step to tracking and improving your ACO's performance. The CMS ACO measure set is a good place to start, along with any measures required by commercial payers. To that list, you may wish to add other measures relevant to your patient population, such as maternity and pediatric care measures.

Implementing a quality improvement process focused on the defined set is a key part of the process. The optimal quality improvement process depends on your ACO's performance gaps, patient population, available resources, and clinical leadership. Regardless of the priorities you set, it is important to use the quality measures to continually monitor progress and identify areas that require attention.

REFERENCES

1. Sawer B, Cox C. How does health spending in the US compare to other countries? *Peterson-Kaiser Health System Tracker*. December 7, 2018. https://www.healthsystemtracker.org/chart-collection/health-spending-u-s-compare-countries. Accessed October 23, 2019.

2. Institute of Medicine. *Crossing the Quality Chasm: A New Health System for the 21st Century*. Washington, DC: National Academies Press; 2001. http://www.nationalacademies.org/hmd/~/media/Files/Report%20Files/2001/Crossing-the-Quality-Chasm/Quality%20Chasm%202001%20%20report%20brief.pdf. Accessed March 22, 2018.

3. McGlynn EA, Asch SM, Adams J, et al. The quality of health care delivered to adults in the United States. *New England Journal of Medicine*. 2003;348(26):2635–2645. doi:10.1056/NEJMsa022615.

4. McCarthy D, How SKH, Fryer AK, Radley DC, Schoen C. *The Commonwealth Fund Commission on a High Performance Health System: Why Not the Best? Results from the National Scorecard on US Health System Performance, 2011*. New York, NY: The Commonwealth Fund; October 2011. http://www.commonwealthfund.org/publications/fund-reports/2011/oct/why-not-the-best-2011. Accessed October 23, 2019.

5. Search quality measures resources. Kaiser Family Foundation web site. https://www.kff.org/tag/quality-measures. Accessed March 22, 2018.

6. Health Services Advisory Group Inc. *2018 National Impact Assessment of the Centers for Medicare & Medicaid Services (CMS) Quality Measures Report*. Baltimore, MD: US Department of Health and Human Services, Centers for Medicare & Medicaid Services; February 28, 2018. https://www.cms.gov/Medicare/Quality-Initiatives-Patient-Assessment-Instruments/QualityMeasures/Downloads/2018-Impact-Assessment-Report.pdf. Accessed March 22, 2018.

7. NQF's history. National Quality Forum website. https://www.qualityforum.org/about_nqf/history/. Accessed April 5, 2018. Refer also to *National Quality Forum Phrase Book: A Plain Language Guide to NQF Jargon*. Washington, DC: National Quality Forum. https://www.qualityforum.org/Field_Guide. Accessed March 15, 2018.

8. The NQF maintains a publicly accessible online database of endorsed measures called the "Quality Positioning System." See: http://www.qualityforum.org/QPS/QPSTool.aspx. Accessed March 15, 2018.

9. Steps for improvement (1): models. Improving Chronic Illness Care website. http://www.improvingchroniccare.org/index.php?p=1:_Models&s=363. Accessed March 8, 2018.

FIVE

Monitoring and Submitting Quality Measures for the Group Practice Reporting Option

Medicare Web Interface

KRIS GATES

Collecting the quality data that an accountable care organization (ACO) generates and reporting it to Medicare are formidable tasks. Kris Gates manages Health Endeavors, a company that conducts this service for many ACOs, including Hackensack Alliance. There are few other companies that perform similar services. Follow Gates's 10 steps to ensure a successful outcome.

Introduction

Collecting, scoring, and reporting quality measures can be daunting tasks for your Medicare ACO. The goal is to collect and document each of the measures throughout the year for your ACO-assigned patient population and then report the ACO quality data in the subsequent year from January to March. In 2019, for example, data for 10 quality measures needed to be collected throughout the year. Reporting is completed by then submitting your data to Medicare's Web Interface (WI) from January to March 2020. Note that what used to be called the group practice reporting option is now the Merit-based Incentive Payment System (MIPS) and using WI as the method of submission.

2019 Web Interface Quality Measures

CARE-2 Falls: screening for future fall risk
PREV-5 Breast cancer screening
PREV-6 Colorectal cancer screening
PREV-7 Preventive care and screening: influenza immunization

PREV-10 Preventive care and screening: tobacco use: screening and cessation intervention

PREV-12 Preventive care and screening: screening for clinical depression and follow-up plan

PREV-13 Statin therapy for the prevention and treatment of cardiovascular disease

MH-1 Depression remission at 12 months

DM-2 Diabetes: hemoglobin A1c poor control

HTN Hypertension: controlling high blood pressure

WI measures must be proactively conducted by your providers and documented in accordance with Medicare guidelines in their paper or electronic health records (EHRs). Failure to successfully report and perform (in applicable years) may result in the reduction of shared savings dollars paid to the ACO.

How Does Your ACO Team Submit Successfully?

Follow our 10 steps to success:

1. Set up Health Endeavors' central data repository for Medicare claims and clinical data. This process requires a clinical data integration plan for each clinic.
2. Decide from the outset of the ACO start date if specialists will complete and/or report the quality measures.
3. Assign every attributed patient to a provider using Health Endeavors' algorithm to ensure financial and quality accountability.
4. Complete the quality metrics for all Medicare fee-for-service patients.
5. Conduct quality measures and workflow training for providers and staff.
6. Use Health Endeavors' Gap Analysis Tool year-round to obtain status of complete, incomplete, and nonperforming measure responses.
7. Send Health Endeavors' secure text message notifications to consumers to alert them of quality care gaps.

8. Use Health Endeavors' Electronic Health Record Application Program Interface Connector to provide actionable quality data at the point of care.

9. Communicate to providers and staff how to access Health Endeavors' Provider Performance Scorecards.

10. Before submission, use Health Endeavors' Optimal Gaps Tool to ensure the best score submission in each measure.

The following will give an overview of each step.

Step 1: Set up Health Endeavors' central data repository for Medicare claims and clinical data. Your ACO needs to get its claims, clinical, and laboratory data integrated into a central repository for gap analysis, performance scoring, and reporting. Your two options to integrate Medicare claims data are (a) monthly Medicare ACO claim and claim line feeds via managed file transfer, or (b) a weekly Medicare Blue Button feed via patient consent in MyMedicare.gov (see figure 5.1). Medicare claims data will prompt the user to see if measures were completed in-network or out-of-network and which measures remain incomplete or have an applicable medical exclusion.

Your options to integrate clinical and laboratory data are (a) Quality Reporting Document Architecture (QRDA), (b) Consolidated Clinical Document Architecture (C-CDA), (c) Fast Healthcare Interoperability Resources (FHIR), or (d) HL7 laboratory data feed (see figure 5.1). Each ACO participant EHR will need to collaborate with Health Endeavors to collect QRDA, C-CDA, FHIR, or a combination of the foregoing into the Health Endeavors (HE) repository. Again, each ACO participant will need a clinical data integration plan with the HE repository as each will have different EHR capabilities.

If using the C-CDA or FHIR process, the best option is to use Health Endeavors' EHR Application Program Interface (API) Connector. Many EHRs already have API technology and it simply takes the HE repository connecting to their API to conduct a C-CDA or FHIR call for data. The EHR API Connector technology also creates a seamless process for the provider team to retrieve a summary of incomplete measures and the ability to notify the consumer of future care gaps via text alerts, which we will discuss in several of the next steps.

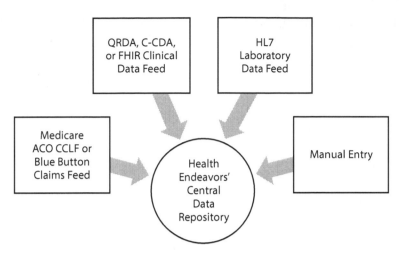

Figure 5.1. Health Endeavors' central data repository can integrate ACO claims, clinical, and laboratory data via a number of different channels: monthly Medicare ACO claim and claim line feeds (CCLFs), Medicare Blue Button feeds, Quality Reporting Document Architecture (QRDA), Consolidated Clinical Document Architecture (C-CDA), Fast Healthcare Interoperability Resources (FHIR), an HL7 laboratory data feed, or manual entry.

We suggest compiling all EHR names and versions from a survey and let the HE repository connect with the EHR vendors in the survey on a consolidated basis as EHRs will pay more attention to large group requests. The ACO team can set up a mass laboratory feed under a master agreement to the central repository.

Once data is fed into the HE repository it will autogenerate complete, incomplete, medically excluded, and complete but nonperforming responses into a gap analysis and generate a text alert to patients at the first of each month for incomplete quality measures.

Claims data is imported into the central repository because it prompts the ACO team as to who performed the measure and where the record is located. Although claims and clinical/laboratory data has been contributed to the repository, manual entry (see figure 5.1) to verify and audit is common during the final submission process.

Step 2: Decide from the outset of the ACO start date if specialists will complete and/or report the quality measures. Many ACOs are moving away from including specialists in their ACO participant list as specialists do not want to be responsible for collecting and reporting WI quality measures. Specialists instead usually report their specialist quality measures under the MIPS program. If you do include specialists in your ACO participant list, then a decision should be made from the outset of the ACO start date what specialists, if any, will collect and report such measures.

Step 3: Assign every attributed patient to a provider using Health Endeavors' algorithm to ensure financial and quality accountability. Use the Health Endeavors patient assignment algorithm to assign every patient to a provider (primary care, mid-level, or specialist, unless determined specialists will not conduct measures) for quality and financial accountability. As you move forward with quality and financial performance analytics, it will be important for each patient to be assigned to one provider (figure 5.2). Therefore, it is critical to decide early on about your specialists. A patient should be assigned to a provider that has made a commitment to financial and quality accountability.

Step 4: Complete the quality metrics for all Medicare fee-for-service patients. Your ACO clinic workflows are not set up to identify which patients are in the Medicare ACO unless the clinic implements Health Endeavors' EHR API Connector, which notifies the clinic upon selection of the patient in the provider's EHR system at the point of care that is patient assignment and attribution. Therefore, initially, every Medicare patient should be treated as if they are in the ACO and the quality measures have been completed for them. Handing out ACO–assigned pa-

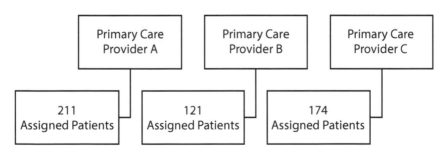

Figure 5.2. Example of assigned patient breakdown after applying Health Endeavors' patient assignment algorithm.

tient Excel lists to clinics will only end up in the circular filing cabinet (i.e., the garbage can) as it doesn't fit into their workflow. Another reason is that patient attribution is updated too frequently to distribute static Excel lists.

Step 5: Conduct quality measures and workflow training for providers and staff. The WI collection and reporting task is daunting because it requires clinical staff to understand each measure and the accepted documentation, method, location, and staff credentials to perform each measure. Make sure your clinical staff understand the following questions:

Who are the clinical staff qualified to perform the quality measure?
What are the data collection requirements?
Where are the physical or telehealth settings that the quality measure may be conducted?
When or in what time frame can the measure be conducted?
How are the quality measures going to be collected and documented?

Regarding the question of "how," each ACO participant clinical staff member should understand the EHR or print workflow for each measure. This means how the quality measure is to be documented in the discrete fields of the EHR so it is included when the QRDA, C-CDA, or FHIR are generated. Failure to use discrete fields results in the inability to easily extract the data electronically.

Step 6: Use Health Endeavors' gap analysis tool year-round to obtain status of complete, incomplete, and nonperforming measure responses. Gap analysis is the automated process of identifying the complete, incomplete, complete with nonperforming, and medically excluded responses autogenerated from the HE repository using claims and clinical data (see figure 5.3).

Your ACO and ACO participant staff will need to check at least monthly as to the progress on their assigned populations. Don't get to the end of the year with only incomplete and nonperforming responses on your progress grid because this will set your final submission to Medicare up for failure.

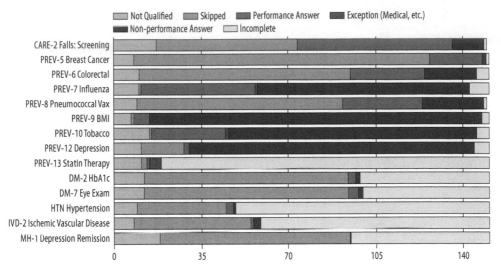

Figure 5.3. Example of a gap analysis reporting on the status of quality measure responses from providers.

Step 7: Send Health Endeavors' secure text message notifications to consumers for quality care gaps. Secure text message notifications to the patient throughout the year of his or her incomplete or nonperforming gaps in care increase the ACO's rate of fully completed measures and high-performance responses (figure 5.4). Ninety-five percent of text messages are opened in minutes, with an 82% turnaround of patients making an appointment in 30 days or less to resolve the care gap. At the same time of text enrollment, have the patient sync their weekly Medicare Blue Button data feeds to replace the monthly ACO claim and claim line feeds.

Step 8: Use Health Endeavors' Electronic Health Record Application Program Interface Connector to provide actionable quality data at the point of care. During the process of setting up the HE repository, Health Endeavors will also set up the EHR API Connector to feed actionable quality data to your EHR using its patient-match technology. When the patient is in the clinic for the visit, the clinical staff opens the patient record in the EHR and the Health Endeavors consolidated patient history with actionable data—including quality, cost, and utilization—will render a display (figures 5.5 and 5.6).

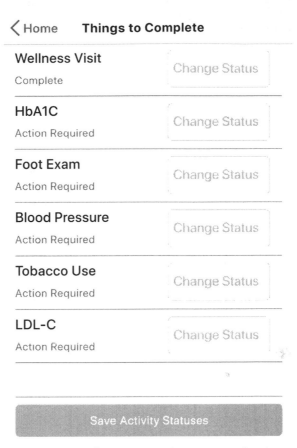

Figure 5.4. Text message notifying patient of care gaps and action required.

Step 9: Communicate to providers and staff how to access Health Endeavors' Provider Performance Scorecards. Performance scoring involves applying the Medicare performance scoring methodology to your central data repository. Medicare provides an ACO score; however, by applying the Medicare performance scoring methodology to your central data repository, your ACO may also obtain location performance scoring (for divisions, facilities, and subfacilities) or individual performance scoring (figure 5.7).

The ACO, divisions, facilities, locations, and individual providers may access their performance via the web by entering their national provider identifier number.

Quality

DM-2 DM with HbA1c > 9 percent (poor control)		Not Applicable
HTN-2 Controlling High BP	✕	**Action Required**
MH-1 Depression Remission		Done
PREV-5 Breast Cancer Screening		Not Applicable
PREV-6 Colorectal Cancer Screening	✕	**Action Required**
PREV-7 Influenza Immunization	✕	**Action Required**
PREV-10 Tobacco Use: Screening and Cessation Intervention		Not Applicable
PREV-12 Screening for Depression and Follow-up Plan	✕	**Action Required**
PREV-13 Statin Therapy	✕	**Action Required**
Care-2 Falls: Screening for Future Fall Risk	✕	**Action Required**
Wellness Visit Done Last 12 Mo	✕	**No - 04/24/2017 - Complete**

Figure 5.5. Health Endeavors' Electronic Health Record Application Program Interface Connector display showing actionable gaps in quality measures of care.

Cost and Utilization

2018 YTD Spend	$20945.80
2018 HCC Benchmark	$16778.70
2018 HCC Benchmark vs 2018 YTD Spend ⊗	**125.00%**
Out of Network Spend*	$16401.07
Office Visits*	03-23-2018;04-16-2018;08-14-2018;10-17-2018;10-19-2018;11-01-2018
Most Visited Provider*	1003808809 MR. SHARAM DANESH MD
Last Wellness Visit* ⊗	**04/24/2017**
Admits* ⊗	1
Readmissions*	0
ED Visits*	0
ED Visits that led to Hospitalizations*	0
CT Scans* ⊗	2
MRI Events*	0

Figure 5.6. Health Endeavors' Electronic Health Record Application Program Interface Connector display showing cost and utilization data.

PREV-5	PREV-6	PREV-7	PREV-8	PREV-9
90%	90%	90%	90%	90%
92.19%	58.78%	29.87%	44.60%	4.26%
100.00%	78.57%	28.21%	36.84%	2.27%
71.43%	65.64%	50.00%	69.57%	2.38%
87.50%	44.44%	38.46%	50.00%	2.13%
80.0%	43.75%	53.85%	72.73%	6.67%

Figure 5.7. Example of a Health Endeavors Provider Performance Scorecard showing a breakdown of ACO scores from Medicare as well as location and/or individual performance scoring.

Step 10: Before submission, use Health Endeavors' Optimal Gaps Tool to ensure the best score submission in each measure. In January, your ACO, if it participated in the ACO program in the prior year, will receive a random sample of approximately 25% of your attributed patients to remit quality measure responses.

Each year Medicare grants 8 to 10 weeks to prepare the final ranked sample quality-response submission. If your ACO has conducted steps 1 to 9 outlined here, your ACO should be ready to click "final submit" within days unless you want to conduct an audit. Not only will your ACO be able to submit within days of receipt of the random sample, your ACO will already know your performance score at the ACO, division, facility, location, or individual provider level prior to submission.

Random sample patients will be grouped by measure with a rank of 1 to 616 or 750. A few comments about ranks:

- Patients may be ranked in some but not all measures.
- Patients are ranked 1 to 616 or 750 in each measure.
- There may be fewer than 616 or 750 if there were not enough patients to fill the measure; for example, your ACO may not have enough diabetic patients that meet the ranking selection process.
- Your ACO is required to complete patients ranked from 1 to 248 consecutively. The patients ranked from 249 to 616 or 750 is the oversample.
- For every skipped patient in a measure, the ACO will need to complete the next consecutive patient (e.g., 249, 250). ACOs may complete all patients in the random sample in each measure and then decide which consecutive patients to remit based on their optimal score.

Health Endeavors' optimal gaps report provides critical information about how many patients in the oversample of each quality measure the ACO should submit to obtain the optimal score (e.g., 248, 414, or 616). Again, if the ACO completes all 616 or 750, then the optimal gaps report provides the number of patients to submit in each measure for the best possible score.

An option for newer ACOs or ACOs that have not completed steps 1 to 9 is to use the HE repository technology to default measures to "not done" or "no diagnosis," to skip if applicable, to complete, or to diagnosis responses not found electronically in the clinical data.

Do All 10 Steps for Success

By completing all 10 steps, your ACO will

- have year-round access to progress and performance;
- have a complete cycle-of-care program, including quality care gaps, to text to patients and prompt them to make any follow-up appointments;
- obtain actionable quality data at the point of care;
- be able to remit its final submission within days of receipt of the rank sample with little to no manual keying of data; and
- know its performance score at all levels of the organization before clicking "final submit."

Repeating the 10 steps for your Healthcare Effectiveness Data and Information Set, Comprehensive Primary Care Plus, and Medicaid quality measure programs will have the same successful results.

SIX

Live Experience of a Quality Measure Validation Audit

MITCHEL EASTON

The Centers for Medicare and Medicaid Services (CMS) periodically audits reported compliance with their quality measures. Mitch describes Hackensack's experience during such an audit. How to prepare and successfully complete the audit are explained in great detail. In the end, the process will make you a more successful accountable care organization (ACO).

Introduction

You are being audited on a sample of . . .

Not unlike receiving a letter from the IRS advising of an audit of your personal tax return, these opening words from CMS notifying your Medicare Shared Savings Program (MSSP) ACO of a pending quality measure validation (QMV) audit are apt to trigger a healthy dose of angst for all of us.

Anxiety can be a powerful motivator. But if you can channel it within a constructive framework of knowledge and understanding, this knee-jerk response can be transformed into a welcomed opportunity for expanded awareness, education, and ultimately a positive change for your ACO.

This chapter covers the process of a QMV audit, including its intended purpose and scope, potential trigger events, and the benefit of maintaining a positive mind-set during the ensuing analysis and your ACO's final response submission to CMS. Most, if not all, of the discussion presented here is based upon the actual QMV audit of Hackensack Alliance ACO that occurred in April and May 2016 and was based on our 2015 group practice reporting option (GPRO) submission. Since it began in April 2012 as a Track 1 ACO with the MSSP, Hackensack Alliance has enjoyed six successive performance years (through PY 2018) of positive gain-sharing, and this has been our only QMV audit experience. While CMS may have slightly modified the QMV process in subsequent years, there is no reason to believe that the core goal and structure have significantly changed. Most importantly, the potential benefits of "lessons learned" remain steadfast.

There is no guarantee that your MSSP ACO will ever be selected for a QMV audit, but the odds do increase with each year of your participation in the program. Chance aside, consciously planning for its eventuality can help ease the impact and burden of getting through it with a positive experience and productive result. No ACO can completely control *if* you get audited, but you can influence *how* you respond to it and embrace it. The goal then is to share the Hackensack Alliance ACO QMV experience with you as part of the overall recipe of "how to be a successful Medicare ACO."

With the recent CMS overhaul of the MSSP embodied in the new Pathways to Success model, there were many new complexities and nuances to consider as the new program commenced on July 1, 2019. It's far too early to know if and how the QMV audit process will be influenced. It's nevertheless reasonable to believe that the core goal of the audit remains the same: to validate the ACO's reporting of quality measures submitted via the CMS Web Interface.

Every journey begins with the first step. Remember the first two helpful rules of the QMV audit:

1. Breathe
2. See rule #1

Quality Measure Validation

A fundamental goal of the annual GPRO survey is to *document* an ACO's effectiveness in monitoring, addressing, and reporting its ability to close clinical care gaps across a pool of specific quality measures. Then it follows that a cardinal goal of QMV is to *verify* the ACO's ability to accurately report the evidence of those gap closures as properly recorded in the clinical documentation (paper chart or electronic health/medical record) of the ACO's attributed population.

Validation: the action of checking or proving the validity or accuracy of something

In short, the GPRO provides the opportunity for ACOs to self-report clinical quality through the lens of specific quality measures on a sample population selected by CMS. QMV provides CMS a vehicle to ensure, to *validate*, that ACOs are fulfilling their obligation to completely and accurately report their submission of clinical quality data via the GPRO. But there is perhaps a less obvious purpose lurking in the haze that accompanies the anxiety of a QMV audit, just waiting to be acknowledged and leveraged: it provides your ACO an opportunity to examine and improve its reporting accuracy through augmented awareness and better education.

Quality and Cost of the Medicare Shared Savings Program

Per CFR 42 §425.10(a), CMS established the Medicare Shared Savings Program to

- promote accountability for a patient population,
- coordinate care and services under Medicare Parts A and B,
- encourage investment in infrastructure,
- redesign care processes for high quality and efficient services, and
- incent higher value care.

It is a gain-/loss-sharing model (dependent upon track or level) that has the potential to financially reward an ACO based on its aggregate performance with respect to delivery of quality care (both process- and outcome-based) and on its efficient, active cost management of its attributed Medicare population. Both performance elements, quality and cost, are compared against CMS benchmarks to determine an ACO's overall performance. However, both elements are interdependent such that neither alone can result in a financial reward for the ACO. Cost efficiencies without quality performance will not be financially rewarded and vice versa.

Table 6.1. Quality domains and their weight in the quality score

Quality source	Quality domain	Quality domain weight (%)
Accountable care organization CAHPS[a] survey	Patient/caregiver experience	25
Claims and group practice reporting option (GPRO) survey	Care coordination and patient safety	25
GPRO survey	Preventive health	25
GPRO survey	At-risk population	25

[a]Consumer Assessment of Healthcare Providers and Systems.

The ACO's performance year report from CMS reflects these two pivotal performance measures: finance and quality. The financial portion reflects the ACO's ability to manage cost by comparing its PY total benchmark expenditures (i.e., CMS's "should cost" amount) against its PY total actual expenditures (i.e., the ACO's actual cost). The quality portion reflects the ACO's quality score against individual quality measure benchmarks. Oversimplified here, a net financial savings is factored by the quality score yielding an amount for joint (CMS and the ACO) gain-sharing in accordance with the particular ACO track or level criteria. The takeaway in this oversimplified explanation is that expenditures and quality are joined at the hip in determining any potential financial reward.

The ACO's composite quality score (delivered as part of the final performance year financial and quality report) is based on data collected across four equally weighted quality domains. The ACO's GPRO quality measure data submitted to CMS constitutes more than 50% of the ACO's quality score (table 6.1). This underscores the importance of the GPRO to the ACO and to CMS, both in terms of accurately reflecting the ACO's effective preventive health and risk-based care and having a very significant influence on any potential financial gain-sharing reward.

Trust, but Verify

The need for a CMS quality measure validation tool for data collected and reported to CMS via the annual GPRO submission can be traced to the fact that the GPRO is inherently a *self-reporting* pathway for every MSSP ACO. CMS auditors do not review and submit data on behalf of an ACO during the GPRO. It is the ACO who is fully responsible for operationally abstracting clinical chart data to support quality measure reporting to CMS through either the web interface directly, or through an authorized third party vendor on behalf of the ACO. This self-reporting context is steeped in an assumption of implicit honesty and trust by CMS that the ACO will report accurately and completely.

The QMV audit is a case of *trust, but verify*. CMS's authority to audit and validate quality data reported by an ACO is anchored in CFR 42 §425.500.

Audit Objectives

The GPRO quality data reported to CMS is subject to a QMV audit. The audit objectives are to

1. determine the accuracy of the performance year data by comparing ACO reported data (GPRO) with available supporting documentation (charts),
2. assist in identifying areas to target for education and outreach, and
3. address reporting anomalies as needed with the ultimate goal of improving future reporting accuracy among all ACOs.

As a condition of participation in the Medicare Shared Savings Program, an ACO selected for audit must participate as directed by CMS. But what determines if an ACO is selected for audit? While CMS reserves the right to audit whenever it deems appropriate to ensure program compliance, it's widely assumed that selection of specific ACOs for the QMV audit is predicated on two general factors:

1. Systematic random selection with the goal of annually validating a representative sample of all ACOs
2. Exceeding trigger event thresholds on submitted GPRO quality data, which might include excessively reported measure skips, exceptions, and/or exclusions

Audit Scope

The Hackensack Alliance ACO QMV audit shared here focused on the 17 quality measures submitted to CMS during the 2015 GPRO survey. A subset of five quality measures was selected by CMS for audit:

> CARE-2 (ACO-13) Falls: screening for future fall risk
> DM-7 (ACO-41) Diabetes: eye exam
> HF-6 (ACO-31) Heart Failure: beta-blocker therapy for left ventricular systolic dysfunction
> MH-1 (ACO-40) Depression remission at 12 months
> PREV-12 (ACO-18) Preventive care and screening: screening for clinical depression and follow-up plan

In the (unlikely) event that one of the chosen five measures did not yield a sufficient beneficiary sample size for audit, an alternate measure was available for selection by CMS:

> CAD-7 (ACO-33). Coronary artery disease: angiotensin-converting enzyme inhibitor or angiotensin receptor blocker therapy— diabetes or left ventricular systolic dysfunction (LVEF < 40%).

For Hackensack Alliance ACO's QMV audit, the alternate measure was not required since the chosen five quality measures yielded suitable sample sizes.

CMS randomly selects a sample of 30 beneficiaries for each of five measures. Thus, 150 beneficiaries (150 ranked measures) were selected for QMV audit from our total 2015 GPRO sample population of 3,936 (3.8%). For all selected beneficiaries, our ACO was required to provide and submit documentation that fully supported the original GPRO submission responses. Fully supportive documentation should be understood to mean copies of the applicable and relevant portions of the beneficiary's clinical chart, including screen snippets of the electronic health record, as required. The goal is to fully substantiate the original GPRO ranked measure response by addressing the following key measure elements (as applicable):

- Diagnosis confirmation or denominator criteria
- Numerator inclusions
- Denominator exceptions
- Denominator exclusions

For a full list of documentation requirements, please see appendix A, "Medical Record Documentation Collection and Submission," at the end of this chapter.

All supporting documentation is then forwarded to CMS (via its contractor) for review and evaluation to determine if the clinical data evidence provided fully supports the original GPRO submission response for each ranked measure being audited. If so, a "CMS match" is declared for that ranked measure. If not, a "CMS mismatch" is declared for that ranked measure. As you might assume, a CMS mismatch is not desirable since it reflects variance between responses submitted via the GPRO versus evidence documented in the clinical record.

Audit Methodology

The QMV audit may have up to three phases. Phase 1 and phase 2 compare the information reported by the ACO's GPRO submission with the supporting documentation submitted as described in the previous section on audit scope. If the supporting documentation does not match what was reported in the GPRO, it is considered a mismatch. During phase 1, eight randomly selected beneficiaries for each audited measure are reviewed. If there are no mismatches identified for a measure, the audit of that measure is considered complete and no further action is taken for that measure (table 6.2). However, if there are mismatches, then the audit progresses to phase 2 for those measures with mismatches. During phase 2, the remaining beneficiaries' supporting documentation is reviewed for each audited measure that did not pass phase 1. If a mismatch rate of greater than 10% between the GPRO quality data reported and the supporting documentation provided for any measure is determined in phase 2, the audit progresses to phase 3. During phase 3 the ACO must provide a

	Mismatch threshold		
	0% discrepancy in phase 1	1%–10% discrepancy in phase 1	>10% discrepancy in phase 2
Phase 1	No further action needed		
Phase 2		✓	
Phase 3			✓

Table 6.2. Evaluation phases of a quality measure validation audit

written explanation for each measure that has a greater than 10% mismatch rate identified in phase 2.

Now that I've finished outlining the structure and incremental evaluation criteria of the QMV audit in general, I'd like to share our specific ACO's audit experience.

A Quality Measure Validation Case Study

On March 11, 2016, Hackensack Alliance ACO enjoyed its final submission to CMS of our 2015 GPRO quality measure submission via our valued and long-time partner vendor, Health Endeavors. As with every prior GPRO survey closure, our ACO exhaled a very audible collective sigh of exhilarated relief and proud accomplishment. The next GPRO was a pleasing and leisurely year away.

On April 7, however, we received CMS notification of our pending QMV audit based upon our 2015 GPRO submission just three weeks prior. We had picked the short straw.

Notification

At the time we first digested the words "You are being audited," we had not yet fully appreciated the first two helpful rules of the impending audit, which I'll reiterate here:

1. Breathe
2. See rule #1

Our ACO would not receive additional details of the QMV audit, including the specific sample population chosen, for an additional two weeks. Nevertheless, the initial notification (and all subsequent communication) was immediately shared with full ACO leadership, the ACO clinical and administrative staff, as well as the corporate and ACO compliance officer. Full transparency and timely communication were key.

CMS contractor Telligen provided a comprehensive and helpful document that included the audit background (authority), objective, scope, methodology, sample population, measures, and timeline to provide a proper response. The priority was to devise a realistic and effective plan of attack:

1. Create a tiger team consisting of key clinical, analytical, and GPRO abstraction staff.
2. Formulate a clear understanding of the QMV audit results document from CMS, including all response requirements and their respective timelines.
3. Identify key tiger team members who will manage the review and response workflow, including data validation, collection of required relevant medical documentation, analysis of inconsistencies found, and authoring the final narrative response to CMS, which may, if appropriate, include a corrective action plan.
4. Await the receipt of the QMV audit sample, which will consist of 30 reported beneficiary measures for each of five quality measures (150 total).
5. Distribute the audit sample for re-abstraction of medical documentation to support the submitted GPRO responses.
6. Aggregate, collate, and submit to CMS the required documentation in strict accordance with QMV instructions.
7. Await the receipt of the QMV audit results. After analysis of the documentation submitted, CMS will prepare a comprehensive QMV audit results document for our ACO that will include a detailed audit mismatch report. Mismatches are those cases where the medical documentation submitted does not adequately support the original GPRO response.

8. Validate the QMV mismatch detail report provided by CMS. Compare the individual mismatch detail report responses against the responses formally submitted via GPRO.
9. Review and analyze fully validated mismatches to understand the nature and number of inconsistencies (mismatches) reported by CMS. Be open to discovering trends that could reflect things like general workflow deficiencies, incomplete or improper understanding of certain measure criteria (especially exceptions and exclusions), and abstractor or data source specific anomalies.
10. If the tiger team concludes that the CMS-reported mismatches are valid, prepare a formal response to CMS that addresses augmented internal controls and/or corrective actions that will be implemented to improve the accuracy of reported information in the future.
11. The response narrative to CMS, including any corrective action plan, should have the full consensus of the tiger team and the entire ACO leadership before being submitted to CMS. The value of a thoughtful, relevant, and comprehensive narrative response cannot be overstated in terms of both satisfying CMS and providing a blueprint for improved internal ACO procedures.

Analysis and Results

CMS (via its contractor, Telligen) provided a complete analysis of all supporting clinical documentation that was previously submitted for each of the 150 QMV audit samples. The official audit results (mismatches) included both summary and detail-level findings. Our QMV audit mismatch summary data is in table 6.3, and the complete audit mismatch detail is provided in appendix B.

These unanticipated results did not imbue pride for us, and a full review of the QMV audit followed. The mismatch detail report confirmed that our ACO truly "earned" these results. Initial review by CMS determined that we had exceeded the 10% trigger threshold of phase 2 for selected measures. In fact, almost 20% of our audit sample

Table 6.3. Quality measure validation audit mismatch summary

Measure	Measure title	Number of mismatches	Mismatch percentage (%)	Audit result phase
CARE-2	Falls: screening for future fall risk	2 of 30	6.7	2
DM-7	Diabetes: eye exam	9 of 30	30.0	2
HF-6	Heart failure: beta-blocker therapy for left ventricular systolic dysfunction	8 of 30	26.7	2
MH-1	Depression remission at 12 months	6 of 30	20.0	2
PREV-12	Preventive care and screening: screening for clinical depression and follow-up plan	4 of 30	13.3	2
Overall results		29 of 150	19.3	

reflected inadequate, improper, or missing clinical documentation to support the recorded GPRO response. The impact on our ACO staff was palpable, but the choice ahead for the tiger team was evident. We could wallow in the disappointment or use this outcome as an opportunity. It was a wake-up call to objectively examine GPRO abstraction workflows (at the systemic level as well as at the individual abstractor level). We identified knowledge gaps of quality measure criteria and created an action plan to improve accuracy, accountability, and knowledge.

Discussion of Analysis and Results

To determine potential root causes of documented mismatches, it was useful to categorize our errors into logical groups or "buckets," where each group could be descriptively characterized by the shared traits of the errors. The high-level grouping also improved our ability to identify potential causes and to recommend specific pathways to resolution and remediation. The overarching goal in all cases was to minimize the likelihood of similar future mistakes. Beyond the initial shock of this unexpectedly poor report card, we were determined to use this unplanned opportunity to *learn* and then to *apply* that knowledge to leverage improvement to our ACO success. Despite our year-over-year success in achieving substantial shared savings since inception (2012), there was still ample room for improvement.

The 29 documented mismatches were distilled into the following general categories, which are not necessarily mutually exclusive:

Errors of Omission and Commission

Without addressing *intent*, which could arguably be worthy of consideration, these errors were the result of an imperfect decision process that concluded supporting evidence was available when it was not or, conversely, supporting evidence was not available when it actually was available.

Errors of Imperfect Knowledge

Perfect knowledge, while highly desirable, typically reflects only an ideal state. But in the real world, human abstractors represent a varied pool of clinical experience, expertise, and judgment. Although the full quality measure specifications were available to every abstractor, the final interpretation and decision-making process during the GPRO is nevertheless sometimes predicated on inadequate, incomplete, or improper knowledge of the individual abstractor.

Errors of Expediency

Human nature often includes an irrational component that can influence behavior. The GPRO is often an anxiety-riddled event, a necessary evil that must be endured, frequently with inadequate and/or competing resources to accomplish the task at hand. Cognitively, we are all too aware of its importance and implications. Nevertheless, the potential influence of *get-it-done-itus* cannot be ignored.

With the above three general error pools in mind, the following specific quality measure mismatch errors are summarized.

1. CARE-2
   a. Denominator exclusion: improper use of medical reason
2. DM-7
   a. Diagnosis confirmation missing
   b. Inadequately specified as "retinal" or "dilated"
   c. Inadequately specified "negative" result

3. HF-6
   a. Missing "LVEF < 40%" or the absence of the characterization of "moderate or severe dysfunction" in the clinical documentation for heart failure
   b. "40%–45%" ejection fraction (EF) in chart does not equal < 40%
   c. Missing diagnosis confirmation
   d. Metoprolol: must be succinate (extended release), not tartrate
   e. Missed a valid denominator exception for medical reason
4. MH-1
   a. Denominator exclusion: assisted living is not equal to permanent nursing home resident
   b. Denominator exclusion: insufficient support for diagnosis of bipolar disorder or for diagnosis of personality disorder
5. PREV-12
   a. Positive depression screening: insufficient or missing positive result
   b. Improper screening tool: not an age appropriate standardized tool
   c. Denominator exclusion: missed a valid denominator exclusion

After reviewing the confirmed mismatch errors found in each of the five measures, some readers may be inclined to conclude that the three chosen error buckets may not be exhaustive enough, or granular enough, or are perhaps too overlapping and nondistinct. But they were nevertheless helpful to us. Each offered a hint on how to address and potentially remediate, with a few key observations and impressions bubbling to the surface:

- Absent or weak evidence was used to support measure compliance, including confirmation of diagnosis.
- Inappropriate evidence was used to support measure compliance.
- Not only was missing or improper evidence used to support measure compliance, but available evidence was also missed to support a valid exclusion that could have been declared.

- Potential existed for stretching the boundary between acceptable and unacceptable supporting documentation.
- Additional education was needed to reinforce a more complete understanding of measure compliance criteria.

Building a Response

Our multidisciplinary ACO tiger team was charged with the responsibility of managing the QMV audit from beginning to end. This included formally acknowledging the QMV audit (both to CMS and local ACO leadership), providing the requested supporting documentation to CMS, reviewing and analyzing the official QMV audit mismatch results report, and providing a formal response to CMS and ACO leadership regarding future corrective actions.

On June 29, 2016, we prepared a formal written response that we believe fully addressed the QMV audit specifically but also addressed key elements and planned actions that would improve its ability to completely and accurately report quality data in the future.

The QMV audit provided an unexpected opportunity to reflect upon internal processes that we assumed were well honed. Although not particularly welcomed initially, the cited deficiencies forced a systematic and thoughtful reassessment that would ultimately be welcomed and beneficial.

Our written response to CMS was structured around the following salient points:

- Transparent acknowledgment of deficiencies cited
- Proposed corrective actions, focused on global and non-measure-related as well as measure-specific
- Pledge to leverage this opportunity for future improvement
- Consensus and support of full ACO leadership

Our ACO's full written response to CMS on August 11, 2016, follows. It is not offered as a prescribed template but rather as an example of what our ACO considered to be a relevant, realistic, and complete response to CMS.

Hackensack Physician-Hospital Alliance ACO LLC (HPHA ACO) is pleased to respond to the 2015 QMV Audit Analysis (prepared on June 29, 2016) provided by CMS to HPHA ACO on July 29, 2016 as part of the PY2015 Financial Reconciliation and Quality Performance Report. This document is submitted to CMS on August 11, 2016 (within the required 15 calendar day response window).

Acknowledgment

HPHA ACO acknowledges and concurs with the audit analysis regarding the following four quality measures cited in the CMS report:

- DM-7: Diabetes: Eye Exam
- HF-6: Heart Failure: Beta-Blocker Therapy for Left Ventricular Systolic Dysfunction (LVSD)
- MH-1: Depression Remission at 12 Months
- PREV-12: Preventive Care and Screening: Screening for Clinical Depression and Follow-Up Plan

Further, HPHA ACO is committed to identifying and addressing key deficiencies, to determine individual and global accountabilities, to promote remediation through augmented education and implementation of corrective action plans (CAP), and to require future periodic reviews to validate that CAPs are achieving the desired results.

Introduction

Shortly after our 2015 QMV Audit was submitted to CMS, an internal analysis of our submitted documentation was conducted due to the high number of mismatches observed. Our internal findings were consistent with the official CMS QMV Audit Report, and thus were promptly presented to HPHA ACO Executive Leadership for discussion, further investigation, planning, and subsequent action. The complete official 2015 QMV Audit Report was shared with HPHA ACO Executive Leadership and full ACO staff (including GPRO abstractors) on August 2, 2016. This document is the product of both our own internal analysis, and of the 2015 QMV Audit Report issued by CMS.

The deficiencies reported, and our approach to remediation, will be presented in two sections: Non-Measure-Specific (Global) Elements and Measure-Specific

Elements. Together, these sections address areas of needed improvement or refocus for both the four specific measures cited above, as well as overall improved data collection and reporting for the broader spectrum of all quality measures.

Non-Measure-Specific (Global) Elements

1. Accountability: Our current abstraction process allows us to specifically identify which GPRO surveyor supplied information for every beneficiary measure data point as the data is recorded, as well as after the fact. The results of this QMV have already been used to identify specific surveyors who appear to inadequately or improperly record GPRO responses in the context of the available medical record data. Identified surveyors will receive targeted and focused remedial training and education. Similarly, during actual GPRO abstraction, the identified abstractor who is linked to the specific data point recorded can be monitored via web portal in near real time.

2. Team-Based GPRO Surveyors: Frequently, a single GPRO surveyor was assigned to abstract data representing a defined beneficiary subpool. As a result, we have determined that the quality of abstraction may vary from surveyor to surveyor based on the individual's education, medical experience, GPRO audit experience, etc. A team approach of two surveyors per team will mitigate these individual variances, with the goal of improved abstraction accuracy and consistency. Our future approach will insure that there is at least one RN as a member of the two-person team. Further, our team-pairing model will insure that a "seasoned surveyor" always accompanies a less experienced abstractor as a teammate.

3. Random Spot Check Validation: During the actual GPRO audit period, we will employ random "spot check" validations of recorded data before upload to QualityNet. These validation checks will not be conducted by the original surveyor-recorder, but rather by independent surveyor to maintain objectivity, insure a more consistent and accurate measure response, and to offer immediate feedback, education, and correction as required. Additionally, HPHA ACO will incorporate "spot check" validation audits throughout the performance year as measure data is collected. Results of these audits will be reported to Executive Leadership and the larger ACO staff to drive improved collection techniques and reporting accuracy on a continuing basis.

4. Enhanced EMR Data Aggregation and Abstraction: HPHA ACO participants include multiple and varied EMR platforms that provide challenges to a consistent and objective data abstraction methodology across diverse systems. Traditionally, this had resulted in a disproportionate amount of manual abstraction. Already underway, and scheduled over the next 6–12 months, additional data warehousing tools will be implemented to facilitate more efficient and accurate measure collection and reporting. While manual abstraction will never be completely eliminated, this enhanced functionality will allow for a lower amount of manual abstraction, and its associated human error component. Surveyors can spend more focused time validating already recorded discrete data, rather than data mining.

5. Quality Measures Education and Abstraction Training: There is no substitute for education and training. Many quality measures are quite straightforward and leave little room for misinterpretation. Other measures are filled with nuances regarding inclusion/exception/exclusion criteria that are less clear to the less experienced surveyor. Historically, HPHA ACO has concentrated quality measures education and GPRO abstraction training just prior to the start of the formal GPRO audit. To augment our current efforts, HPHA ACO will conduct mandatory education and training for all current and candidate ACO abstractors. We will start with 6-week education/training intervals. Non-ACO employees (identified as "ACO Champions") who are part of our participating medical practices will also be invited to attend. Our educational resources will include the following CMS approved and provided documents:

a. Accountable Care Organization 2015 Program Analysis Quality Performance Standards Narrative Measure Specifications guide
b. 2015 GPRO [Disease Specific] Supporting Documents workbooks
c. GPRO [Disease Specific] Quality Measure Quick Reference Guides

Measure-Specific Elements
DM-7: Diabetes: Eye Exam
The deficiencies noted include insufficient documented support to confirm a diagnosis of diabetes (2 out of 30) and insufficient documented support for a retinal or dilated eye exam by a qualified optometrist or ophthalmologist during the measurement (or prior) year (7 out of 30). HPHA ACO concurs with

this analysis, and we have identified the two abstractors responsible for recording the patient measures. Additional discussion, education, and training will be provided to the two identified abstractors to gain insight regarding interpretation of the measure and to promote a more accurate understanding of the measure criteria. Educational resources will include the *Accountable Care Organization 2015 Program Analysis Quality Performance Standards Narrative Measure Specifications Guide* and the *2015 GPRO DM Supporting Documents v6.0 Workbook.*

HF-6: Heart Failure: Beta-Blocker Therapy for LVSD

The deficiencies noted include insufficient or contrary documented support for LVEF of less than 40%, or qualitative documentation for "moderate" or "severe" LVSD (5 of 30); documented support for a non-qualifying form of metoprolol (1 out of 30); insufficient documented support to confirm a diagnosis of HF (1 out of 30); and insufficient documented support to confirm a prescribed beta blocker (1 out of 30). HPHA ACO concurs with this analysis, and we have identified the four abstractors responsible for recording the patient measures. Additional discussion, education, and training will be provided to the four identified abstractors to gain insight regarding interpretation of the measure and to promote a more accurate understanding of the measure criteria. Educational resources will include the *Accountable Care Organization 2015 Program Analysis Quality Performance Standards Narrative Measure Specifications Guide,* and the *2015 GPRO HF Supporting Documents v6.0 Workbook.*

MH-1: Depression Remission at 12 Months

The deficiencies noted include insufficient documented support for a denominator exclusion based on permanent nursing home resident, active diagnosis of bipolar disorder, or active diagnosis of personality disorder (3 out of 30) and improper support for a denominator exclusion (permanent residence in assisted nursing facility is not equivalent to permanent residence in nursing home) (1 out 30). HPHA ACO concurs with this analysis, and we have identified the two abstractors responsible for recording the patient measures. Additional discussion, education, and training will be provided to the two identified abstractors to gain insight regarding interpretation of the measure and to promote a more accurate understanding of the measure criteria. Educational resources will include the *Accountable Care Organization 2015 Program Analysis Quality Performance Standards Narrative Measure Specifications Guide*, and the *2015 GPRO MH Supporting Documents v7.0 Workbook*.

PREV-12: Preventive Care and Screening: Screening for Clinical Depression and Follow-Up Plan

The deficiencies noted include insufficient documented support for a positive depression screen result (2 out of 30); insufficient documented support for the use of an age appropriate standardized depression screening tool (1 out of 30); and insufficient documented support confirming an active diagnosis of bipolar disorder prior to the measurement period to support a claimed denominator exclusion (1 out of 30). HPHA ACO concurs with this analysis, and we have identified the abstractor responsible for recording the patient measures. Additional discussion, education, and training will be provided to the identified abstractors to gain insight regarding interpretation of the measure and to promote a more accurate understanding of the measure criteria. Educational resources will include the Accountable Care Organization 2015 Program Analysis Quality Performance Standards Narrative Measure Specifications guide, and the 2015 GPRO PREV Supporting Documents v6.0 workbook.

Summary

HPHA ACO appreciates the opportunity to respond to the 2015 QMV Audit Analysis provided by CMS. It has highlighted four specific areas of needed improvement; however, we believe that it has also afforded us an opportunity to examine and improve our data collection and reporting efforts across all quality measures. HPHA ACO will not squander this opportunity to review, modify, and improve our understanding of each measure, as well our ability to accurately report chart documentation supporting measure compliance (or meeting appropriate exception and exclusion criteria).

Response Document Approval

This 2015 QMV Response Document has been reviewed and approved by the HPHA ACO President and CEO (Morey Menacker, DO), and by the HPHA ACO Chief Medical Officer (Edward Gold, MD). It is authorized for submission to CMS on August 11, 2016.

Point of Contact Regarding This Document

To confirm receipt of this document, or to address any questions regarding this document, please direct all inquiries to:

Mitchel Easton, ACO CMS Liaison, ACO Data Analyst

Hackensack Physician-Hospital Alliance ACO LLC (A1006)

In the weeks that followed our QMV response submission to CMS, the ACO received a formal acknowledgement of receipt from CMS (via its QMV subcontractor). Beyond that, there was no additional communication from CMS regarding the need for any added clarification or amplification of our formal written response. Our working assumption was that our response fully acknowledged and addressed all cited deficiencies.

Final Recommendations

While there is no assurance that any other (or every other) ACO's QMV audit experience will mirror ours exactly, it's reasonable to posit generalities that can be drawn from our specific experience that will be applicable to other MSSP ACOs, both past and future. By sharing Hackensack Alliance ACO's experience and the generalities that arose from it, it's our earnest hope that it will relieve or reduce anxiety and sow the seeds for using the QMV audit as a humbling and positive learning experience. So, what potential general lessons can be distilled from our experience that may serve as one more relevant ingredient for you to lead a more successful ACO?

- *Relax*: The QMV audit is an anxiety-producing event. Breathe, and keep breathing.
- *Be humbled*: Regardless of your ACO's past success, and despite how well honed you believe your data abstraction, validation, and reporting workflows may be, allow for improvement that comes with close scrutiny by an objective third party (CMS).
- *Acknowledge*: Promptly acknowledge receipt of CMS's letter advising of an impending QMV audit.

- *Be transparent*: Promptly advise ACO leadership, and other corporate leadership as appropriate, of the upcoming audit. Keep all stakeholders regularly informed of milestone dates, ongoing progress, and any obstacles to progress.
- *Form a tiger team*: Create a team consisting of representatives from administrative, clinical, analytical, GPRO abstractor staff, and quality measure subject matter experts. The tiger team will lead the overall effort to fully understand all QMV audit requirements, generate and manage a response plan (including key milestone dates), formulate and submit a formal response to CMS, and keep the broader ACO leadership apprised of progress.
- *Use a critical view and be open to discovering trends*: As you objectively investigate mismatches, be open to discovering patterns that emerge that may indicate weaknesses in workflow, knowledge, or larger systemic information flows. Include the "human factors" in your review and consideration process.
- *Adapt to your findings and apply corrections*: Based on specific findings, identify potential improvement activities that fundamentally address the causes of identified deficiencies. Implement those corrective activities that will improve processes and accuracy over the long-term. Be willing to dismantle and rebuild teams and methodologies as appropriate.
- *Stay positive*: There is nothing "fun" about a QMV audit. But with the right attitude, it can be an opportunity to faithfully examine current processes, highlight and reinforce those that serve the ACO well, and discover those that might need to be reengineered to achieve improved results.

Finally, in his book *Project Retrospectives: A Handbook for Team Reviews* (Dorset House, 2001), Norman Kerth articulated his "prime directive," which has some relevance here, particularly with respect to the human element and its contribution to any process and associated outcomes.

The Prime Directive: Regardless of what we discover, we understand and truly believe that everyone did the best job they could, given what they knew at the time, their skills and abilities, the resources available, and the situation at hand.

Regardless of how much technology is a part of your overall GPRO data abstraction collection and reporting effort, it's we humans who perform and oversee the validation process for reporting quality measure care gap closures as evidenced in the patient's medical record. It is we humans who endorse and certify that the submitted data is complete, accurate, and true. An ideal goal is to never make a mistake. A practical goal is to allow daylight to gently expose our mistakes in an accepting atmosphere that values and supports improvement over perfection. Our best today can be even better tomorrow.

APPENDIX A

Medical Record Documentation Collection and Submission

CARE-2 (ACO-13) Falls: Screening for Future Fall Risk
Numerator Inclusions
- Documentation indicating the patient received screening for future fall risk (patient's fall history)

Denominator Exceptions
- Documentation in the medical record to indicate if there was a medical reason why the patient was not screened for future fall risk

DM-7 (ACO-41) Diabetes: Eye Exam
Confirm Diagnosis/Denominator Criteria
- Documentation confirming the patient has a history of diabetes during the measurement period or year prior to the measurement period (claims information cannot be used to confirm the diagnosis of diabetes as claims are the original source of the diagnosis sampling)

Numerator Inclusions
- Dated office note, letter, eye exam report indicating the patient had a retinal or dilated eye exam by an ophthalmologist/optometrist

OR
- Dated office note, letter, eye exam report indicating the patient had a negative retinal eye exam (no evidence of retinopathy) by an ophthalmologist/optometrist during the year prior to the measurement period

HF-6 (ACO-31) Heart Failure: Beta-Blocker Therapy for Left Ventricular Systolic Dysfunction (LVSD)
Confirm Diagnosis/Denominator Criteria
- Documentation confirming the patient has an active diagnosis of heart failure at any time in the patient's history up through the last day of the measurement period (claims information cannot be used to confirm the diagnosis of heart failure as claims are the original source of the diagnosis sampling)

AND
- Documentation indicating the patient has left ventricular systolic dysfunction (i.e., LVEF less than 40% or documented as moderate or severe and can have occurred any time in the patient's history up through the last day of the measurement period)

Numerator Inclusions
- Dated medication list indicating the patient is on beta-blocker therapy or dated office visit note indicating the patient is on beta-blocker therapy (bisoprolol, carvedilol, or extended-release metoprolol succinate are the *only* beta-blockers allowed for this measure)

Denominator Exceptions
- Documentation in the medical record to indicate if there was a medical, patient, or system reason why the patient was not prescribed beta-blocker therapy

MH-1 (ACO-40) Depression Remission at Twelve Months
Confirm Diagnosis/Denominator Criteria
- Documentation confirming the patient has a diagnosis of major depression or dysthymia during the denominator identification period, December 1, 2013, to November 30, 2014 (claims information cannot be used to confirm the diagnosis of major depression or dysthymia as claims are the original source of the diagnosis sampling)

AND
- Documentation indicating the patient had a Patient Health Questionaire-9 (PHQ-9) administered during the denominator identification measurement period (index date) between December 1, 2013, and November 30, 2014 and a score greater than 9 (including date and value)

Denominator Exclusions
- Documentation in the medical record to indicate the patient had a denominator exclusion (permanent nursing home resident > 1 year any time before the start of the measurement period or an active diagnosis of bipolar

disorder or active diagnosis of personality disorder during the denominator identification period or during the assessment period)

Numerator Inclusions
- Documentation indicating the patient had a PHQ-9 administered during the measurement assessment period and a score less than 5 at 12 months (+/− 30 days) of the index date (including date and value)

PREV-12 (ACO-18) Preventive Care and Screening: Screening for Clinical Depression and Follow-Up Plan
Denominator Exclusions
- Documentation indicating the patient has an active diagnosis of depression or bipolar disorder diagnosed prior to the first day of the measurement period.

Numerator Inclusions
- Documentation indicating the patient was screened for clinical depression using an age appropriate standardized tool and the screen was *negative* including name of tool

OR
- Documentation indicating the patient was screened for clinical depression using an age appropriate standardized tool and the screen was *positive* including name of tool

AND
- Documentation indicating the patient received a follow-up plan regarding depression (discussion of the plan must be specified as an intervention that pertains to depression and must be documented on the date of the positive screen)

Denominator Exceptions
- Documentation in the medical record to indicate if there was a medical or patient reason why the patient was not screened for clinical depression

(Alternate Measure) CAD-7 (ACO-33) Coronary Artery Disease: Angiotensin-Converting Enzyme (ACE) Inhibitor or Angiotensin Receptor Blocker (ARB) Therapy—Diabetes or Left Ventricular Systolic Dysfunction (LVEF < 40%)
Confirm Diagnosis/Denominator Criteria
- Documentation confirming the patient has an active diagnosis of coronary artery disease or history of cardiac surgery at any time in the patient's history up through the last day of the measurement period (claims information cannot be used to confirm the diagnosis of coronary artery disease as claims are the original source of the diagnosis sampling)

AND

- Documentation indicating the patient has diabetes and/or left ventricular systolic dysfunction (i.e., LVEF less than 40% or documented as moderate or severe and can have occurred any time in the patient's history up through the last day of the measurement period)

Numerator Inclusions

- Dated medication list indicating the patient is on ACE inhibitor or ARB therapy or dated office visit note indicating the patient is on ACE Inhibitor or ARB therapy

Denominator Exceptions

- Documentation in the medical record to indicate if there was a medical, patient, or system reason why the patient was not prescribed ACE inhibitor or ARB therapy

APPENDIX B

Quality Measure Validation Audit Mismatch Detail

CARE-2

Audit case	Element	ACO answer	Audit determination	Rationale for mismatch
2	Fall risk screening	Medical reason	No	The documentation provided did not support a medical reason to not screen the patient for fall history.
7	Fall risk screening	Medical reason	Yes	The documentation provided did not support a medical reason to not screen the patient for fall history. The documentation provided indicated the patient or caregiver was queried about the patient's fall history.

DM-7

Audit case	Element	ACO answer	Audit determination	Rationale for mismatch
1	Diagnosis confirmation	Yes	Yes	
	Eye exam	Yes	No	The documentation provided does not indicate eye screening for diabetic retinal disease, identified by a retinal or dilated eye exam by an optometrist or ophthalmologist performed during the measurement period or a negative retinal exam performed by an eye care professional during the year prior to the measurement period.

2	Diagnosis confirmation	Yes	Yes	
	Eye exam	Yes	No	The documentation provided does not indicate eye screening for diabetic retinal disease, identified by a retinal or dilated eye exam by an optometrist or ophthalmologist performed during the measurement period or a negative retinal exam performed by an eye care professional during the year prior to the measurement period.
10	Diagnosis confirmation	Yes	No	The documentation provided did not indicate the patient had a documented history of diabetes during the measurement period or year prior to the measurement period.
	Eye exam	Yes	N/A	
11	Diagnosis confirmation	Yes	Yes	
	Eye exam	Yes	No	The documentation provided does not indicate eye screening for diabetic retinal disease, identified by a retinal or dilated eye exam by an optometrist or ophthalmologist performed during the measurement period or a negative retinal exam performed by an eye care professional during the year prior to the measurement period.
15	Diagnosis confirmation	Yes	Yes	
	Eye exam	Yes	No	The documentation provided does not indicate eye screening for diabetic retinal disease, identified by a retinal or dilated eye exam by an optometrist or ophthalmologist performed during the measurement period or a negative retinal exam performed by an eye care professional during the year prior to the measurement period.
16	Diagnosis confirmation	Yes	Yes	
	Eye exam	Yes	No	The documentation provided does not indicate eye screening for diabetic retinal disease, identified by a retinal or dilated eye exam by an optometrist or ophthalmologist performed during the measurement period or a negative retinal exam performed by an eye care professional during the year prior to the measurement period.
23	Diagnosis confirmation	Yes	Yes	
	Eye exam	Yes	No	The documentation provided does not indicate eye screening for diabetic retinal disease, identified by a retinal or dilated eye exam by an optometrist or ophthalmologist performed during the measurement period or a negative retinal exam performed by an eye care professional during the year prior to the measurement period.

Audit case	Element	ACO answer	Audit determination	Rationale for mismatch
24	Diagnosis confirmation	Yes	Yes	
	Eye exam	Yes	No	The documentation provided does not indicate eye screening for diabetic retinal disease, identified by a retinal or dilated eye exam by an optometrist or ophthalmologist performed during the measurement period or a negative retinal exam performed by an eye care professional during the year prior to the measurement period.
29	Diagnosis confirmation	Yes	No	The documentation provided did not indicate the patient had a documented history of diabetes during the measurement period or year prior to the measurement period.
	Eye exam	Yes	N/A	

HF 6

Audit case	Element	ACO answer	Audit determination	Rationale for mismatch
2	Diagnosis confirmation	Yes	Yes	
	Left ventricular systolic dysfunction (LVSD)	Yes	No	The documentation provided did not indicate the patient had LVSD (current or prior left ventricular ejection fraction (LVEF) less than 40% or documented as moderate or severe).
	Beta-blocker	Yes	N/A	
6	Diagnosis confirmation	Yes	Yes	
	LVSD	Yes	No	The documentation provided did not indicate the patient had LVSD (current or prior LVEF less than 40% or documented as moderate or severe). The patient's ejection fraction was 40%–45%.
	Beta-blocker	Yes	N/A	
9	Diagnosis confirmation	Yes	Yes	
	LVSD	Yes	Yes	
	Beta-blocker	Yes	No	The documentation provided indicated the patient was prescribed metoprolol; however, it did not indicate that it was extended-release.
13	Diagnosis confirmation	Yes	Yes	
	LVSD	Yes	No	The documentation provided did not indicate the patient had LVSD (current or prior LVEF less than 40% or documented as moderate or severe). The patient's ejection fraction was 68%.
	Beta-blocker	Yes	N/A	

15	Diagnosis confirmation	Yes	Yes	
	LVSD	Yes	No	The documentation provided did not indicate the patient had LVSD (current or prior LVEF less than 40% or documented as moderate or severe). The patient's ejection fraction was 45%.
	Beta-blocker	Yes	N/A	
21	Diagnosis confirmation	Yes	Yes	
	LVSD	Yes	No	The documentation provided did not indicate the patient had LVSD (current or prior LVEF less than 40% or documented as moderate or severe).
	Beta-blocker	Yes	N/A	
23	Diagnosis confirmation	Yes	No	The documentation provided did not indicate the patient had an active diagnosis of heart failure.
	LVSD	Yes	N/A	
	Beta-blocker	Yes	N/A	
26	Diagnosis confirmation	Yes	Yes	
	LVSD	Yes	Yes	
	Beta-blocker	Patient reason	Medical reason	This is not considered a mismatch and is provided for education only. The documentation provided is inconsistent with a patient reason for not prescribing beta-blocker therapy. The patient had a biventricular implantable cardioverter defibrillator, which is a medical reason for not prescribing beta-blocker therapy.
27	Diagnosis confirmation	Yes	Yes	
	LVSD	Yes	Yes	
	Beta-blocker	Yes	No	The documentation provided did not support that the patient was prescribed or is currently taking beta-blocker therapy.

MH-1

Audit case	Element	ACO answer	Audit determination	Rationale for mismatch
4	Diagnosis confirmation	Denominator exclusion	No	The documentation provided did not support the presence of denominator exclusion for disqualification from this measure (permanent nursing home resident, active diagnosis of bipolar disorder, active diagnosis of personality disorder). The patient resides in assisted living, which is not considered a permanent nursing home for the purposes of this measure.
	Index Patient Health Questionaire -9 (PHQ-9)	N/A	N/A	
	PHQ-9 > 9	N/A	N/A	
	Assessment PHQ-9	N/A	N/A	
	PHQ-9 < 5	N/A	N/A	

7	Diagnosis confirmation	Denominator exclusion	No	The documentation provided did not support the presence of denominator exclusion for disqualification from this measure (permanent nursing home resident, active diagnosis of bipolar disorder, active diagnosis of personality disorder).
	Index PHQ-9	N/A	N/A	
	PHQ-9 > 9	N/A	N/A	
	Assessment PHQ-9	N/A	N/A	
	PHQ-9 < 5	N/A	N/A	
17	Diagnosis confirmation	Denominator exclusion	No	The documentation provided did not support the presence of denominator exclusion for disqualification from this measure (permanent nursing home resident, active diagnosis of bipolar disorder, active diagnosis of personality disorder).
	Index PHQ-9	N/A	N/A	
	PHQ-9 > 9	N/A	N/A	
	Assessment PHQ-9	N/A	N/A	
	PHQ-9 < 5	N/A	N/A	
21	Diagnosis confirmation	Denominator exclusion	No	The documentation provided did not support the presence of denominator exclusion for disqualification from this measure (permanent nursing home resident, active diagnosis of bipolar disorder, active diagnosis of personality disorder).
	Index PHQ-9	N/A	N/A	
	PHQ-9 > 9	N/A	N/A	
	Assessment PHQ-9	N/A	N/A	
	PHQ-9 < 5	N/A	N/A	
23	Diagnosis confirmation	Denominator exclusion	No	The documentation provided did not support the presence of denominator exclusion for disqualification from this measure (permanent nursing home resident, active diagnosis of bipolar disorder, active diagnosis of personality disorder).
	Index PHQ-9	N/A	N/A	
	PHQ-9 > 9	N/A	N/A	
	Assessment PHQ-9	N/A	N/A	
	PHQ-9 < 5	N/A	N/A	
28	Diagnosis confirmation	Denominator exclusion	No	The documentation provided did not support the presence of denominator exclusion for disqualification from this measure (permanent nursing home resident, active diagnosis of bipolar disorder, active diagnosis of personality disorder).
	Index PHQ-9	N/A	N/A	
	PHQ-9 > 9	N/A	N/A	
	Assessment PHQ-9	N/A	N/A	
	PHQ-9 < 5	N/A	N/A	

Audit case	Element	ACO answer	Audit determination	Rationale for mismatch
15	Depression screening	Yes	Yes	
	Positive screen	Yes	No	The documentation provided did not support the result of a positive depression screen.
	Follow-up plan	Yes	N/A	
20	Depression screening	Yes	No	The documentation provided did not support completion of depression screening using an age-appropriate standardized tool.
	Positive screen	No	N/A	
	Follow-up plan	Yes	N/A	
22	Depression screening	Yes	Yes	
	Positive screen	Yes	No	The documentation provided did not support the result of a positive depression screen.
	Follow-up plan	Yes	N/A	
24	Depression screening	Yes	Denominator exclusion	The documentation provided indicated the patient had an active diagnosis of bipolar disorder prior to the measurement period.
	Positive screen	Yes	N/A	
	Follow-up plan	Yes	N/A	

SEVEN

Ready, Risk, Reward

Building Successful Two-Sided Risk Models

BRENT HARDAWAY, ELYSE PEGLER, AND BRYAN SMITH

Since the inception of the Medicare Shared Savings Program in 2012, most accountable care organizations (ACOs) have been in Track 1, which meant if they saved money, they could have potentially shared the savings with the Centers on Medicare and Medicaid Services (CMS) on a 50/50 basis if their quality score was perfect. Track 1 carries no downside risk. But CMS wants all ACOs to eventually assume downside risk, which means sharing part of your losses with CMS. Consequently, after two, three-year terms in Track 1, ACOs must now switch to a track with downside risk. Brent, Elyse, and Bryan explain the tracks that comply with providing both upside potential and downside risk. The older Tracks 1+, 2, 3, and Next Generation and the newer Basic and Enhanced tracks are considered. The authors show in exquisite detail how to prepare for the transition to downside risk and how to prosper under the Basic and Enhanced tracks.

Introduction

Fee-for-service pressures are pushing health systems to pursue alternative payment options for economic survival. The pressures originate from payment penalties and reimbursements that are increasingly tied to performance on measures of quality, satisfaction, and cost management. Continuing the movement away from fee-for-service and toward value-based reimbursement, alternative payment models (APMs) create new opportunities for your health care system and payers. You can now work together on improving health for patients and better managing costs. It is essential for health systems to understand what is driving the continuum-wide cost and quality outcomes included in their risk arrangements. Together you can continuously identify and prioritize gaps in care and build and implement the core capabilities needed to succeed in the rapidly increasing number of APMs.

With nationwide growth in accountable care organizations and other APMs, such as bundled payment models, the continued development and expansion of models that support value-based care is inevitable. Today there are more than 900 active public and private ACOs in the United States, covering more than 32 million people (1). While Medicare contracts represent about 30% of the covered lives in ACOs, commercial contracts represent nearly 60% and Medicaid covers about another 10%–12% (1). The enactment of the Medicare Access and CHIP Reauthorization Act (MACRA), which was passed by a bipartisan vote, also creates positive incentives for clinicians to move away from fee-for-service in favor of APMs. In addition, APMs are starting to see success, as Medicare ACOs have documented a savings of approximately $2 billion and reported measureable improvements in quality (1).

The Medicare Shared Savings Program (MSSP) requires ACOs that have participated in the program since its inception nearly six years ago to either move to a two-sided risk model or drop from the program altogether after 2018. MACRA also reinforces two-sided risk models by rewarding clinicians for participating in advanced alternative payment models (Advanced APMs) to earn even more financial rewards in exchange for taking on risk related to patient outcomes. Additionally, a recent survey of ACOs suggests that nearly half have at least one contract that requires downside risk today. Furthermore, nearly half of ACOs are planning to participate in future at-risk arrangements (2).

It has been well documented that there has been less success in some ACO models. For example, even though the Pioneer ACO program generated $304 million in savings over the first three performance years and half the ACOs generated shared savings payments, the number of Pioneer ACOs dropped from 32 in 2012 to 9 in 2016 (though it's important to note that many, if not most, of these ACOs moved to the Next Generation model or to an MSSP model). These ACOs dropped out of the Pioneer program for a number of reasons, including problems with prospective attribution and the difficulty of being benchmarked against yourself. For example, if an ACO had already been working on population health management, there was less room for improvement and therefore less opportunity for shared savings. These issues still exist but are being addressed in different ways. Ultimately, Pioneer moved to MSSP because there is less risk and to Next Generation because it offered more regional benchmark adjustments and hierarchical condition category (HCC) coding opportunities.

The Next Generation ACO model was developed in an attempt to address many of the issues that were identified, such as regional benchmarking, risk scoring, infrastructure payments, performance-based payments, and risk corridors. However, even the Next Gen ACOs have seen issues, as evidenced by the number of participants that dropped out after CMS went through a rebasing of HCC targets.

As you contemplate whether or not to move into, or move further into, risk-based contracts, consider that there continues to be evidence that ACOs are meeting the goals that have been set out for them—specifically, making improvement in the Triple Aim (improved patient experience, improved health of the population, and reduced total cost of care). CMS recently announced strong Next Generation ACO results with 32 of the 44 participants earning shared savings, saving Medicare $129 million.

As value-based APMs succeed and progress, government and commercial payers are driving providers toward contracts that require them to take more accountability for outcomes that are increasingly tied to varying levels of financial risk. This has left the health care industry at a critical juncture in time, as two-sided risk arrangements for providers are becoming more prevalent. Now more than ever, you have to take a risk by assuming a financial stake in the outcome of the population's care.

While CMS was the early leader in this area, commercial payers now make up the majority of covered lives for alternative payment arrangements. They, too, see the benefits of engaging in two-sided risk contracts with providers to drive costs down and improve quality. In fact, more than half of ACOs report bearing the same levels of financial risk in their commercial and Medicaid contracts as their accountable care contracts with Medicare (2). In discussions with the five largest commercial insurers, Premier Inc. learned that each payer is aggressively transitioning to value-based arrangements that include provider downside risk. The payers have begun to implement this policy in select markets. Furthermore, major employers are adopting two-sided risk models to control health care costs as well as removing intermediaries and aligning incentives to share savings between employees, providers, and the company.

Commercial payers report lower cost and utilization trends, greater patient experience and quality outcomes, and higher rates of preventative care as a result of their value-based accountable care and bundled payment programs. For example, in interviews with UnitedHealthcare, they noted that their accountable care program has seen an 8%–12% medical cost advantage over the market and 14% fewer emergency room visits. Cigna reports seeing 86% of their ACOs perform equal to or better than market on medical cost trends, and 57% performed better on quality measures.

Many APMs require providers to assume a minimal level of risk, known as upside models, where a provider can share in savings with a payer but will not be responsible for losses if they do not meet their goals. The only economic risk is not recovering the investment costs to build the APM through shared savings. Two-sided risk models take APMs to the next level. They engage providers to be accountable for both upside and downside financial risk. They provide stronger incentives to better manage overall costs to avoid losses. Finally, if successful, the ability to earn greater shared savings provides greater rewards for the ACO. These arrangements are also attractive to physicians participating in Advanced APMs through MACRA's Quality Payment Program. Consequently, providers that are not considering or preparing for two-sided risk models could lose market share to competitor organizations, payers, and venture capitalists, such as Aledade and Privia. These organizations are taking advantage of today's market dynamics by building their own relationships with high-value physician networks in order to pursue potentially more lucrative two-sided risk arrangements.

Effective two-sided risk arrangements offer access to powerful bonus rewards and freedom from regulations that undermine innovation.

They represent a smart business choice for providers to ensure continued economic viability in today's risk-based health care environment. The challenge for you as a provider is determining your readiness for assuming greater levels of risk and prudently managing that risk. Some ACOs report that they will not be ready to assume two-sided risk for a number of years. Other ACOs are concerned about ever being ready to assume downside risk (2).

As you negotiate risk contracts, be aware of the issue of duplication of infrastructure. Make sure that there is savings in overhead for the end consumer by making sure that if your health system provides care coordination, that the payer lowers their administrative fees to the employer group. As health systems and ACOs build up their infrastructure, make sure that the payer makes the appropriate adjustments in pricing.

While two-sided risk arrangements are more challenging and require very specific clinical, technical, and administrative capabilities across the continuum, if executed properly, they create opportunities for providers and clinicians to leverage greater financial incentives to improve care delivery practices. At the same time, payers and employers reduce expenses by paying for fewer unnecessary services, fielding fewer health care complications, and achieving better patient outcomes. As these models continue to take hold, you must be well prepared and skilled at assessing and managing risk before diving into these contracts with public and/or private payers. Just as the reward is greater, so is the financial risk. Even though most two-sided risk arrangements can limit the downside risk, accurately assessing readiness is critical to success.

Levels of Risk and Types of Alternative Payment Models

As seen in figure 7.1, one-sided risk models provide the ability for providers to share any savings they achieve with a payer, relative to a spending target, without accepting downside risk. Health care providers that are new to value-based payment should first engage in a one-sided risk APM to build their core capabilities and learn how to manage the health of a population. For those still eligible to do so, participation in a no-downside Medicare APM is a perfect opportunity to learn how to man-

ONE-SIDED RISK	TWO-SIDED RISK	CAPITATION/GLOBAL PAYMENT
Reward: Typically payer and provider split shared savings 50/50 **Risk:** None, except recovery of the investment to the alternative payment model **Risk mitigation:** Minimum savings rate, caps **Key capabilities:** Effective population health IT and care management system	**Reward:** Payer and provider split shared savings between 60/40 and 75/25 **Risk:** Shared loss **Risk mitigation:** Minimum savings rate, minimum loss rate, stop-loss, reinsurance **Key capabilities:** Effective population health IT and care management systems	**Reward:** Provider owns 100% of savings **Risk:** 100% loss **Risk mitigation:** Stop-loss, reinsurance **Key capabilities:** Effective population health IT and care management systems, benefit redesign, risk assessment, including actuarial projections, utilization management, systems, and in-network steerage

Lower   **LEVEL OF FINANCIAL RISK**   Higher

Figure 7.1. Risk continuum of alternative payment models. Courtesy of Premier Inc.

age care, use unblinded claims data as an important tool for success, and acclimate physicians to risk arrangements.

After gaining experience and developing capabilities to manage populations under a one-sided risk APM, many organizations decide to implement "two-sided risk with guardrails." This model places limitations on an organization's downside risk. For example, an organization with a 5% cap on downside risk and a per capita expenditure of $10,000 per beneficiary could lose a maximum of $500 per beneficiary if they exceed the spending target. An example of this is MSSP Track 1+, as listed in table 7.1. Two-sided risk models start with limited risk sharing and move to greater levels of risk depending on provider readiness. With additional risk comes additional opportunities for reward. While Medicare has several two-sided risk models with a variety of risk-sharing options, on the commercial side, providers and payers negotiate specific terms. Structured appropriately, two-sided risk arrangements can limit downside risk and provide even more upside potential than is available in one-sided arrangements. The more recent two-sided risk models in

Table 7.1. Examples of alternative payment models relative to level of financial risk

Payer	One-sided risk	Two-sided risk	Capitation	Other
Medicare Fee-for-Service	Pathways to Success Basic Tracks A & B[a] MSSP Track 1[b] Comprehensive ESRD Care (CEC) One-Sided Risk Model Oncology Care One-Sided Risk Model	Pathways to Success Basic Tracks C, D & E[a] Pathways to Success Enhanced Track[a] MSSP Track 1+[b] MSSP Track 2[b] MSSP Track 3[b] Next Generation ACO Model[c] CEC Two-Sided Risk Model[c] Oncology Care Two-Sided Risk Model[c] Comprehensive Care for Joint Replacement Track 1[c]	Next Generation ACO Model (option)[c]	Bundled Payments for Care Improvement— Advanced[c] CPC+ Track 1[c] CPC+ Track 2[c]
Medicare Advantage (MA)	Negotiated between MA plan and providers	Negotiated between MA plan and providers	Negotiated between MA plan and providers	Joint venture Provider-sponsored health plan
Commercial Health Plan	Negotiated between plan and providers	Negotiated between plan and providers	Negotiated between plan and providers	
Medicaid			Massachusetts Oregon Maryland Global Budget	Arkansas Bundled Payment

[a] Anticipated to have had an open application period in 2019.
[b] Replacements for the programs have been announced and no new entrants are allowed.
[c] Advanced APM, which allow clinicians and providers to earn even more rewards in the Quality Payment Program in exchange for taking on risk related to patient outcomes.

CMS's Pathways to Success are shown in table 7.2, as well as the risk versus reward comparison of each track.

Capitation or global payment, an Advanced APM that most providers are not yet prepared for, is the end goal on the risk spectrum for providers and payers. In most cases, full capitation or global payment models put your organization at risk to meet financial and clinical thresholds for all of the services it provides.

Table 7.2. Comparison of Basic Track and Enhanced Track risk versus reward characteristics

	Basic Track's Glide Path					Enhanced Track (Track 3) (risk/reward)
	Level A & Level B (one-sided model)	Level C (risk/reward)	Level D (risk/reward)	Level E (risk/reward)	Level E (risk/reward)	
Shared savings (once minimum savings rate is met or exceeded)	First dollar savings at a rate up to 40% based on quality performance, not to exceed 10% of updated benchmark	First dollar savings at a rate of up to 50% based on quality performance, not to exceed 10% of updated benchmark	First dollar savings at a rate of up to 50% based on quality performance, not to exceed 10% of updated benchmark	First dollar savings at a rate of up to 50% based on quality performance, not to exceed 10% of updated benchmark	First dollar savings at a rate of up to 50% based on quality performance, not to exceed 10% of updated benchmark	No change. First dollar savings at a rate of up to 75% based on quality performance, not to exceed 20% of updated benchmark
Shared losses (once minimum loss rate is met or exceeded)	N/A	First dollar losses at a rate of 30%, not to exceed 2% of ACO participant revenue capped at 1% of updated benchmark	First dollar losses at a rate of 30%, not to exceed 4% of ACO participant revenue capped at 2% of updated benchmark	First dollar losses at a rate of 30%, not to exceed the percentage of revenue specified in the revenue-based nominal amount standard under the Quality Payment Program capped at 1 percentage point higher than the benchmark nominal risk amount (e.g., 8% of ACO participant revenue in 2019–2020, capped at 4% of updated benchmark)		No change. First dollar losses at a rate of 1 minus final sharing rate, with minimum shared loss rate of 40% and maximum of 75%, not to exceed 15% of updated benchmark

Source: Final rule creates pathways to success for the Medicare Shared Savings Program [fact sheet]. Centers for Medicare and Medicaid website. December 21, 2018. https://www.cms.gov/newsroom/fact-sheets/final-rule-creates-pathways-success-medicare-shared-savings-program. Accessed December 27, 2018.

While understanding financial risk is important, there is more to risk than just the payback. As you increasingly take on downside risk through more sophisticated APMs, you also need to factor in other levels of risk, including the impact of changes in utilization on provider volume and profitability, quality and cost performance targets, and ensuring the technical elements of a contract match population and circumstances (3).

Market Dynamics and Opportunities for Two-Sided Risk

Market dynamics and new payment policies in today's health care industry are driving providers toward two-sided risk arrangements and presenting greater savings splits, the ability to retain high-value physicians as part of MACRA, and the opportunity to achieve higher payments in markets with high utilization and cost rates. However, providers that aren't preparing to take advantage of these opportunities risk losing market share to competitor organizations, payers that are organizing narrow networks, and savvier consumers with increasing involvement in their care decisions.

For instance, CMS is pushing approximately 200 MSSP Track 1 ACO participants that have reached their six-year mark and are entering the final year of their second Track 1 agreements to move into two-sided risk or leave the program. Further, MACRA's Quality Payment Program incentivizes providers to take on two-sided risk by offering clinicians who participate in Advanced APMs the opportunity to earn lump sum bonuses of 5% on their Medicare payments if at least 25% of their Part B payments and 20% of all Medicare patients are from an Advanced APM in 2019, and avoid the downside risk of the Merit-based Incentive Payment System. Therefore, health care organizations engaging in two-sided risk models are appealing to clinicians, making talent easier to retain. Organizations that are not in Advanced APMs risk losing clinicians to competitors that are engaging in these models. This can be a particular issue in markets where competition for qualified medical talent is fierce and health systems may need to offer a range of highly competitive salaries, relocation dollars, signing bonuses, and opportunities for a wide range of APM incentives in order to attract and retain top talent (4).

As discussed earlier, there are additional structural improvements that need to be made to the Next Generation model in order for it to be more appealing to more health systems as they move further into risk taking. Premier Inc., for example, is advocating for CMS to make the following modifications:

- Allow for true primary care capitation within ACO models, such as a set per-beneficiary-per-month payment.
- Allow multiple choices of incentives, such as infrastructure payments, performance-based payments, or capitation, instead of just one choice as it is today.
- Provide greater stability in ACO models and ease the burden associated with implementing waivers.
- Give attribution and financial reconciliation preference to longitudinal, total-cost-of-care models and reward APM entities participating in multiple risk-based models (because model overlap impacts the financial performance of providers who participate in multiple risk models).
- Improve the accuracy of measuring ACO savings by adjusting financial benchmarks to remedy problems with the current approaches, which raise the bar for successful ACOs every year and disadvantage low cost regions as well as providers who are the dominant provider in the region.

While your organization must possess specific capabilities to be successful in two-sided risk models, you must also operate in markets where the macro dynamics are favorable. Providers in high-utilization, high-cost markets stand to gain the most under two-sided risk models. For example, in South Florida, annual Medicare per capita costs range between $16,000 and $17,000 per Medicare beneficiary, compared to the national average of about $9,700 per beneficiary per year. Thus, there is more opportunity to better manage care in these markets with more bandwidth to lower costs, which translates into the potential for greater shared savings payments. But as health care providers better manage these populations' health, per capita dollar amounts are beginning to drop significantly, primarily due to reductions in the unnecessary use of health care services. Therefore, the cost reduction targets will continue to be lowered over time, which means providers, even in these initially high-cost markets, will need to work harder to achieve objectives.

Timing for taking advantage of these macro dynamics is essential. Many providers have lost market share to local competitors that have created risk-bearing entities in high-use, high-cost markets before they were able to do so. Venture capital–based companies are taking advantage of these market dynamics and organizing primary care physicians into independent practice associations, clinically integrated networks, or ACOs while contracting with payers to capitalize on shared savings opportunities. These companies are building ACOs without hospitals and simply view hospitals as cost centers. You need to be aware of this happening in your market and start preparing now by considering the competitive risks of a local venture capital–backed physician network entering your market. The greater number of independent physicians, the greater the risk in a market. Hospitals and health systems that aren't benefitting from these models are losing revenue without the benefit of financial offsets (i.e., shared savings arrangements with payers) if provider competitors are engaged in APMs in their market with commercial and/or government payers. This is because of the utilization reductions that will happen *to* rather than *with* these health systems by APM-engaged competitors and their payer partners.

Additionally, many payer organizations have adopted narrowed networks of health system partners based on cost and quality outcomes, forcing health systems to compete for payer contracts that require mission alignment and expect improved population health outcomes (5) as well as acceptance of two-sided risk arrangements. This movement is supported by the primary care attribution process that is required in most APM arrangements. In other words, as payers increasingly turn to two-sided risk contracts to better manage costs, they may opt to leave providers that aren't prepared to meet financial challenges out of the network in order to offer lower premiums, improve quality performance, increase operating margin, and achieve medical loss ratio targets.

It is imperative for you to prepare for and address these competitive pressures by thoroughly assessing your market and entering into prudent risk arrangements now to take advantage of high per capita costs before they decline and to retain high-value clinicians. For two-sided risk models, the cost savings opportunities are even greater, especially for those in high-cost, high-utilization markets.

Five Capabilities Needed to Succeed in Two-Sided Risk Models

In Premier Inc.'s work with health systems in more than 200 markets across 40 states, we have identified critical factors for planning and implementing a successful transition to value-based payment and increasingly taking on risk.

To create an effective two-sided risk arrangement, you first need to assess your readiness and ability to manage risk, define success, and strategically map the operational capabilities needed to achieve that success. It is important that as you engage in APM arrangements you carefully scale up the level of risk you take on. This includes making sure that before you take on two-sided risk, your health system has already established a risk-bearing entity so that participating providers have experience and the organization has implemented the foundational capabilities needed to assume greater accountability for a defined population. Foundational capabilities include having highly engaged C-suite and physician leadership, systematic assessment and administration of risk arrangements, measurement and reporting systems to track and drive improvement, a highly engaged network of high-value primary care providers, and demonstrated ability to coordinate care across the continuum.

It is also important that as you consider greater financial risk with a payer, you conduct an internal and external risk assessment to determine the potential upside and downside from a financial perspective. This is central to determining the likelihood of success in two-sided risk arrangements. It must also be recognized that more advanced capabilities will be required to expand into and succeed at effective two-sided risk APMs.

Health systems pursuing two-sided risk models in partnership with Premier Inc. are focusing on the following five key capabilities to achieve success.

Aligned Strategy, Leadership, and Infrastructure

A successful two-sided risk arrangement requires aligned and effective C-suite, administrative, and physician leadership as well as compensation incentives from the governance entity that oversees the entire enterprise to the physician groups that participate. This means strategic planning to ensure that clinicians and providers are rewarded for efficient and high-quality care but also for access. C-suite leaders and physicians should all be at the table to discuss payment options to ensure alignment and determine an agreed upon, shared infrastructure across risk contracts. In addition, you must define who oversees leadership and management of the arrangement as well as who has ownership and accountability for assessment, implementing, monitoring, and improving APM operations. This includes involving primary and specialty care leaders to ensure they are committed to invest in the success of the two-sided risk arrangement.

One of the most significant oversights in managing risk deals is that the providers are often not brought into the negotiations and, more often, not told of the deal structure. This oversight can leave millions of dollars on the table. According to one study, providers who went at risk for a majority of their patients and had a thorough knowledge of their advanced risk contracting structure were able to reduce their average cost of care for 95% of all patient visits. Those with no real risk obligation and no knowledge of two-sided risks generated financial losses of approximately $42,000 per physician per year (6)—big dollars that can quickly add up to ruin in a two-sided model.

A key consideration for two-sided risk is ensuring providers are aware of the key drivers for return on investment and making sure those metrics are included in the arrangement and individual incentives. When payment options are understood and agreed to by leadership, administrative staff, and clinicians, participants involved with contributing to the APM contract are more apt to better coordinate care across the continuum and implement patient risk stratification, rising risk identification, and care management capabilities that need to be scaled, integrated, and coordinated across populations for two-sided risk models to be successful.

Optimized Execution of Risk Arrangements

To do well in two-sided risk arrangements, you should have a managed care department (or consultative assistance) that is well versed in negotiating two-sided risk contracts. Keys to successful negotiations include effectively sharing accurate and timely claims data across the continuum with all stakeholders, setting realistic and attainable financial targets, tasking providers with meeting specific metrics that have clear definitions, and ensuring terms and conditions are standardized across the network.

Two-sided risk contracts must also consider market factors, such as whether the population at risk is large enough and if the benchmark expenditure rate is high enough based upon actuarial review. It is important for two-sided risk models to have at least 20,000 covered lives to properly spread the risk and balance high-cost outlier cases. Provider factors such as patient panel size are also important; at least 30% of the panel should be in the risk arrangement in order to influence behavior.

Lastly, your health system must be prepared to deal with the impact of lower volume as a result of fewer emergency room visits and fewer inpatient admissions from the population covered by the at-risk contract. There are some levers that can be pulled to help ameliorate the downside, such as small increases in commercial rates, reducing overhead expenses, and using data to help increase in-network utilization and therefore improve market share.

Establishment of a Narrowed High-Value Provider Network

Narrowed high-value provider networks that reach beyond primary and preventive care must be developed to include all the other medical services that may be needed to provide high-quality, cost-effective outcomes. The key here is to bring hospitals, specialists, rehabilitation centers, behavioral health providers, hospice, and post-acute care providers into the network together. With the success of current APMs and in light of future Quality Payment Program requirements, these providers are already being driven toward Advanced APMs, creating an opportunity to bring more clinicians on board with aggressive care management efforts that steer patients toward their in-network services.

If your health system is taking on two-sided risk, you must establish provider participation criteria to evaluate performance across the continuum, determine action plans, and share results with referring providers. Without dependable post-acute providers collaborating with an ACO and acting as an extension of the health system with shared goals, the inconsistency and unpredictability in care can result in increased readmissions, unnecessary or misuse of care, and unfavorable patient outcomes (7). For instance, a *New England Journal of Medicine* study found that for patients hospitalized with congestive heart failure in 2008, Medicare paid about $2,500 in the 30 days after discharge for each patient who received home health care, as compared to $10,700 for those admitted to a skilled nursing facility and $15,000 for those cared for in a rehabilitation hospital (8). With cost differentials like these at stake, two-sided risk contracts demand networks of aligned providers to enable steering to the most cost-effective care setting and also to the most effective providers within that setting.

This requires a renewed emphasis on narrowing the network by analyzing claims and clinical data to identify appropriate use of high-quality providers. Lower performers should be asked to move into a separate network that is not taking on downside risk, if possible. Community partners, social services, and behavioral health providers should also be included to help address social determinants of health. You must then work with selected providers on care redesign efforts, such as sharing care plans and clinical notes to ensure follow-up appointments with primary care physicians, monitoring provider performance, confirming pharmacy compliance, and sharing and analyzing performance data and referral patterns to ensure continuous improvement.

Clinical Integration across Providers and Risk Contracts

Of critical importance is the need for clinicians to have access to information about their patients and the care their patients may have received outside their network so that they can develop, share, and keep track of each patient's care plan. In addition, it is imperative for providers to participate in the development of and abide by established care delivery models. This requires a commitment to care standardization as well as a coordinated care management structure that integrates all populations that are at risk, thereby developing economies of scale necessary for both capital and operating costs.

An effective care management structure is enabled by a technology platform that identifies high-risk and emerging-risk populations, provides access to patient information, and supports the flow of patient services across care management teams. The care management system must also manage the use of high-cost services across the continuum to avoid taking a loss in a two-sided risk arrangement. This is more difficult in a Medicare ACO where directing patients to a network provider must be limited to sharing provider performance information so that patients retain provider choice. In two-sided risk arrangements with Medicare Advantage plans, providers can work with the payer to build in much stronger in-network utilization incentives for patients, such as through benefit design.

Robust Information Management and Analytics

Robust population health and data management entails the use of strategically selected actionable, predictable, and comparable health information technology capabilities to support the clinical and administrative aspects of care with the goal of improving health outcomes. It requires resources to (a) integrate measures across contracts to focus efforts, (b) evaluate and benchmark the effectiveness and return on investment of clinical interventions, (c) establish interoperability between providers to exchange clinical data and to manage and prevent leakage, (d) and integrate clinical electronic health record data with payer claims information.

Two-sided risk arrangements provide opportunities to negotiate with payers to ensure the payer shares robust adjudicated claims data for the population attributed in a risk arrangement in a timely manner. Claims data is typically held by payers, but it can help at-risk providers tremendously to understand hidden areas of inefficiency, such as unfilled prescriptions or a provider with a propensity for ordering too many inappropriate imaging tests, which may not be obvious from the electronic health record alone (9).

Integrating claims data with clinical information also allows the at-risk health system to tap into more mature predictive analytics capabilities to risk-stratify patients and intervene appropriately as well as support workflows that can direct providers participating under payer risk arrangements toward standardized, appropriate, and evidence-based care pathways. Additionally, provider organizations can use this information to identify high-performing clinicians to partner with, which is vital for developing narrow networks specific for payer two-sided contracts and ensuring the greatest opportunity for success under these arrangements.

Conclusion

It is imperative for your health system and associated providers to build effective key capabilities, gain experience, and achieve success with a one-sided risk APM model before pursing and engaging in a two-sided risk model with a government or commercial payer. However, you must take a methodical approach to assessing readiness for risk to avoid jumping into a two-sided risk model too soon; ensure your organizations are well prepared for the risks in order to attain the rewards. Additionally, clinicians and providers that do not take on two-sided risk may miss out on valuable opportunities: greater savings, lower utilization and per capita costs, better quality and outcomes, attracting and maintaining top clinicians talent, and more-satisfied patients. As you move into two-sided risk contracts, the keys to success are ensuring incentives are aligned (including compensation), performance and processes are standardized and being optimized, market conditions are ripe, a narrow and committed network is developed, robust population health data and analytics are implemented, and effective new care delivery models are well established.

REFERENCES

1. Muhlestein D, Saunders RS, McClellan MB. Growth of ACOs and alternative payment models in 2017. *Health Affairs* blog. June 28, 2017. doi:10.1377/hblog201 70628.060719.

2. de Lisle K, Litton T, Brennan A, Muhlestein D. The 2017 ACO survey: what do current trends tell us about the future of accountable care? *Health Affairs* blog. October 4, 2017. doi:10.1377/hblog20171021.165999.

3. Spector JM, Studebaker B, Menges EJ. *Provider Payment Arrangements, Provider Risk, and Their Relationship with the Cost of Health Care.* Schaumburg, IL: Society of Actuaries; October 2015.

4. Daly R. Physician recruitment competition spreads to urban areas: analysis. *HFM Magazine.* February 2016.

5. Somashekhar S, Cha AE. Insurers restricting choice of doctors and hospitals to keep costs down. *Washington Post.* November 20, 2013.

6. Basu S, Phillips R, Song Z, Bitton A, Landon B. High levels of capitation payments needed to shift primary care toward proactive team and nonvisit care. *Health Affairs.* 2017;36(9):1599–1605.

7. Premier Inc. *Inpatient & Beyond: The Post-Acute Care Conundrum.* Charlotte, NC: Premier; 2016. https://www.premierinc.com/downloads/16222_PR_PAC_one -pager_V6.pdf. Accessed November 3, 2019.

8. Mechanic R. Post-acute care: the next frontier for controlling Medicare spending. *N Engl J Med.* 2014;370(8):692–694. doi:10.1056/NEJMp1315607.

9. Weissman JS, Millenson ML, Haring RS. Patient-centered care: turning the rhetoric into reality. *Am J Manag Care.* 2017;23(1)e31–e32.

EIGHT

Post-Acute Care

A Key Consideration for an Accountable Care Organization

ANDY EDEBURN

Post-acute care (PAC) is usually defined as services provided by skilled nursing facilities, long-term acute care hospitals, inpatient rehabilitation facilities, and home health agencies. In reality, it may not be quite that simple. The economic incentives for PAC facilities are often different from that for accountable care organizations or hospitals. In an insightful presentation, Andy explains how best to utilize the services of PAC facilities to benefit the overall health care system.

Introduction

With the advent of the Affordable Care Act and the national awakening to value-based thinking, many health care organizations across the country have recently sought to better leverage the expanding role of post-acute care and evaluate not only its quality and efficiency but also consider improved ways to partner with post-acute providers as part of the broader continuum. If you're exploring thinking around an accountable care organization (ACO), you must absolutely consider how you will approach post-acute care. There is wide variation in performance and outcomes among PAC providers of similar services, outcome data is inconsistent across post-acute settings, and there is considerable overlap among the various post-acute venues. For you, post-acute represents a key area of opportunity for both quality and cost savings.

What Is Post-Acute Care?

While there is a range of interpretations around PAC, it is generally viewed as "a range of medical care services that support the individual's continued recovery from illness or management of a chronic illness or disability." Post-acute care typically encompasses services provided after a hospital stay, although some of these services may be ordered via physician's order without a preceding hospital stay. It's important for you to note that post-acute is not a specific place, nor is it a "continuum of services." Post-acute is a rough grouping of specialized care settings designed to treat patients based on specific conditions or diagnoses. While some post-acute settings have some similarities, they are not all the same and they are not always interchangeable.

There are four major post-acute settings.

Home Health Agencies

Home health care encompasses a wide range of health care services that are provided in the home after an illness or injury. Common home health services include wound care, IV therapy, serious illness management, and therapy. The focus of home health is to foster improved health and independence in a home-based setting. A nurse or therapist, depending on the patient's needs or plan of care, typically delivers home health services. Aides are often deployed in the home to support these service needs. Most patients access home health following an acute hospital discharge or via a primary care physician order. For your patients to qualify for home health, they must have an intermittent skilled service or therapy need and they must be homebound.

Skilled Nursing Facilities

Skilled nursing facilities (SNFs)—more commonly referred to as nursing homes—offer a range of services for your patients who require 24/7 medical oversight but do not require hospital-level care. SNF-level care is also sometimes called "subacute care" or "transitional care." A hospital-based skilled nursing unit is typically licensed as an SNF. Common SNF services include therapy and rehabilitation, complex medical care, IV therapy, post-operative infection management, and similar needs. SNFs work to stabilize and restore functional capability to discharge the patient to home or a lower level of care. Some of your patients discharged to an SNF can transition to long-term care service, which is also often provided in nursing homes. Most SNF patients are admitted after hospital discharge. To qualify for Medicare-covered (and typically Medicare Advantage–covered) skilled services in an SNF, a patient must have spent three preceding days in an acute hospital.

Inpatient Rehabilitation Facilities

Inpatient rehabilitation (sometimes also called "acute rehabilitation") is a highly specialized setting that provides intensive rehabilitation and therapy services (more than three hours per day) to patients that require hospital-level care and must ideally be seen by a physician daily. Typical inpatient rehabilitation patients include individuals with traumatic brain or spinal cord injury, stroke or a major cerebrovascular event, and other complex neurologic or orthopedic issues. Nearly all are admitted following an acute hospital discharge and their admission is contingent on evaluation and approval of a physiatrist.

Long-Term Acute Care Hospitals

Long-term acute care hospitals (LTACHs) encompass highly specialized settings that provide intensive medical management and rehabilitation of highly complex patients that require acute, hospital-level care and must ideally be seen by a physician daily. Typical LTACH patients include individuals with complex pulmonary illness requiring a mechanical ventilator and weaning from it. LTACHs additionally manage multiple complexities, substantial wound management, infectious disease, and multiple IV management. LTACH patients are most commonly admitted after hospital discharge. To qualify for Medicare payment, the Centers for Medicare and Medicaid Services (CMS) necessitates that an LTACH patient requires ventilator weaning or have been in an acute intensive care unit for at least three days during the preceding hospital stay.

Post-Acute Payment and Reimbursement

Medicare or Medicare Advantage pays for most post-acute services. At present, each post-acute setting has its own distinct reimbursement system. There is some degree of commercial payment in certain venues, but it is usually a minor payer.

Much of the variation associated with post-acute care (referenced earlier and explained in greater detail here) is driven by these various payment systems, and your particular circumstance is also likely to offer considerable variation. You are going to discover there are historically few criteria to guide acute hospital discharge planning regarding the "right" post-acute setting for a patient after discharge. A patient who might be managed in a skilled nursing facility might also be cared for via home health. The same may be true for a patient in an inpatient rehabilitation facility or a skilled nursing facility. While some screening tools have been developed and tested over the last decade to inform these placement decisions, no specific approach has been required or adopted by CMS. As a result, most hospitals rely on patient choice, physician advice, and—too often—old habits. These may create significant challenges for you.

Another issue with these "site-specific" payment systems is that they incent post-acute providers to maximize volume. By way of example, SNFs are paid on a per diem basis. Thus, they are incented to maximize length-of-stay and, as an industry, have learned to optimize their payment within this framework. While this is ideal for the SNF provider, it is an enormous financial issue for you. Home health, while not paid in the same way, has also learned how to optimize its revenue over the last several years via operational performance and broad interpretation of the qualification requirements. It's important to note that fiscal year 2019 and 2020 changes to the skilled nursing and home health payment systems are seeking to address some of these historical issues, but volume as the primary motivator for post-acute payment remains.

Given these behaviors and a desire to collapse post-acute payment into one system (rather than the four current systems), CMS was ordered, via the Improving Medicare Post-Acute Care Transformation

Payment Model Features	PAC Unified PPS Goals
• Common unit of service (i.e., a stay or episode) with a patient characteristic risk-adjustment system • Payment adjustment to reflect lower costs in HHA settings • Separate payments for routine and therapy services and for non-therapy ancillary services such as drugs • Outlier policies for unusually high-cost stays and unusually short stays	• Payments would be based on patient acuity rather than the PAC setting • Providers would have fewer incentives to selectively admit some patients over others because payment would track patient resource needs better

Figure 8.1. Post-acute care (PAC) site-neutral payment model features. HHA = home health agency.

(IMPACT) Act of 2014, to study the potential of a site-neutral or "unified" payment system for post-acute care. The results of the study and follow-up analysis determined that such a system would be viable and could be implemented by 2021 (figure 8.1).

Site-neutral payment would represent a substantial paradigm shift for much of the post-acute industry. While long-term acute care hospitals and inpatient rehabilitation facilities have been historically paid via an episodic model, the amounts they would receive under a site-neutral system are likely to be lower. SNF providers, while used to per diem thinking, would have to shift to an episodic model that will emphasize much shorter lengths of stay than they are historically used to. For hospitals and health systems, who own these assets, the shift in payment carries similar financial and operational impacts. CMS has not yet fully decided on the where, when, and how to implement such a system, but it is important for you to understand that it is a topic under discussion.

Post-Acute Care Quality

Historically, data about post-acute care quality and performance has been fairly limited. Knowledge and understanding of providers was often tied to patient experiences, discharge planner perceptions, and general marketplace opinions. Over the last several years, and with the advent of the IMPACT Act, CMS has taken many steps to improve both the quantity and depth of information that will be available to you about post-acute care quality.

While some states may provide limited quality information about PAC providers, CMS uses a five-star rating system to rank them. SNFs have operated under this model for many years, and you will find a depth of data about SNFs within the system, including staffing, quality, and inspection results. Home health has also operated under a similar system that encompasses quality performance data. This information is available online via Medicare's public-facing website. Five-star rankings are also available for inpatient rehabilitation facilities. As a result of the IMPACT Act, post-acute quality data has been steadily improving over the last three years and new quality measures are scheduled to emerge through 2020. For SNFs in particular, the advent of new claims-based measures informs an SNF value-based purchasing system tied to avoidable readmissions.

These improved assessment measures offer an important resource not only for consumers but also for you, as you are seeking to better understand potential post-acute care partners.

Why Is Post-Acute Care Important?

Post-acute utilization represents a significant component of Medicare spending in the United States, accounting for nearly $60 billion in 2016. PAC spending has more than doubled since 2001. On average over the last several years, more than 40% of Medicare fee-for-service acute discharges end up in some kind of post-acute care. Given that so many patients go to post-acute (figure 8.2), they represent a key focus area for you, regardless of your organization's strategic orientation—population health/value-based or fee-for-service.

Post-Acute Care and ACOs

Because PAC is a Part A–covered service, all Medicare ACOs (and similar organizations in value-based environments) have a direct risk for post-acute spending or behavior. As such, these organizations should be

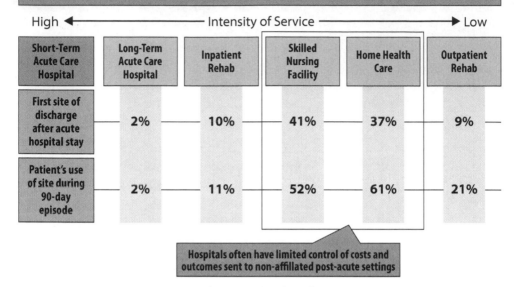

43% of Medicare Beneficiaries Are Discharged from Acute Hospitals to Post-Acute Care					
High ◀——————— Intensity of Service ——————▶ Low					
Short-Term Acute Care Hospital	Long-Term Acute Care Hospital	Inpatient Rehab	Skilled Nursing Facility	Home Health Care	Outpatient Rehab
First site of discharge after acute hospital stay	2%	10%	41%	37%	9%
Patient's use of site during 90-day episode	2%	11%	52%	61%	21%

Hospitals often have limited control of costs and outcomes sent to non-affiliated post-acute settings

Figure 8.2. Post-acute care is the key to bending the cost curve. Courtesy of MedPAC

concerned about PAC spending, much of which is exacerbated by the variability associated with post-acute care.

According to a 2013 study by the Institute of Medicine, post-acute represents the greatest area of variability in health care spending—more than 70% (figure 8.3). By way of comparison, variation for diagnostic testing or acute care is 14% and 27%, respectively. This wide variation means there is a wide risk range associated with post-acute costs, and most health care organizations agree that less risk is always better. As such, paying attention to post-acute spending in a value-based environment is absolutely critical.

Given the volume of patients that historically use post-acute care and the spending associated with it, many ACOs look immediately to post-acute as a means of controlling costs and improving outcomes. Early adopting, proactive ACOs have worked to evaluate and engage capable post-acute providers to define appropriate use, establish performance

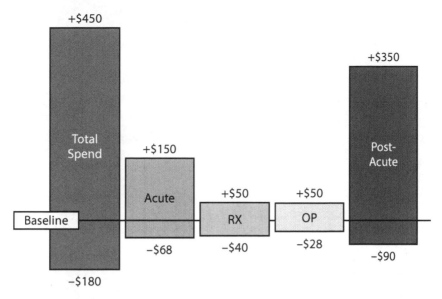

Figure 8.3. Post-acute care is the most variable component of Medicare spending.

expectations, and partner for clinical integration. The ultimate focus of this effort is not only to improve outcomes but also manage spending. This should be a key line of thinking for you as well.

You might ask: why don't I just move all of my patients to the lowest-cost PAC setting? It's a valid question. Some organizations have done exactly that—sought to reduce all of their post-acute use to the least expensive option (which is typically home health). While this approach might work for some patients, it's important to note that it doesn't work for all patients. In a value-based environment, one of the guiding strategies is "appropriate use of sub-specialties." You can't manage every patient in primary care, and you can't use one specialist to address the needs of complex patients. Post-acute is much the same. Complex patients will require specialty care, and in many instances, the best post-acute setting for the patient is the one specifically designed for that patient. Sending a patient to what looks like the lowest-cost option may, in fact, prove to be much more expensive for you in the long run.

Post-Acute Alignment Isn't Obvious

For many acute-centric organizations, the historical alignment with post-acute has been typically tactical or transactional—acute discharge planners or case managers (and sometimes physicians) drive post-acute placement with specific providers or contacts at those organizations. As such, these acute/post-acute relationships have emerged and largely remained based on habit and historical behaviors. You're likely to discover that these will be in conflict with broader strategic needs of the ACO. For instance, you may decide that you want to align strategically with a network of five skilled nursing facilities that have been identified as high quality and agree to work with you around quality and performance improvement. Your strategic intention must first overcome the historical habit of discharge planners who will refer to any post-acute provider—even those that may not be part of your network. Overcoming these sorts of behaviors is discussed in greater detail next.

Post-Acute Can Be First Key Step Outside the Hospital Walls

While all health care is local, the national shift toward "continuums of care" and greater integration with other community-based health care and service organizations is inevitable. For American health care to survive increasing expectations and decreasing payment, it must learn to work collaboratively with other providers to ultimately achieve the Triple Aim of better care, better quality, and lower cost.

Directing patients to community providers and engaging with community providers are not the same thing. Given the immediacy of acute and post-acute relationship, learning to work more closely with post-acute organizations outside the traditional walls is a logical first step for you in connecting with the broader array of community providers. Many organizations across the country have used their post-acute "lessons learned" to build stronger ties to behavioral health, improve management of end-stage renal disease populations, and better engage around the social determinant issues that drive much of our health care spending.

Strategic Thinking around Post-Acute Care

As you start thinking about developing a strategy around post-acute care, it's important to first understand where you and your organization currently stand. There is no one consistent or "ideal" strategy for post-acute engagement. The approach will depend on a number of things. For instance, are you still predominantly a fee-for-service environment or are you more heavily value-based in an ACO or in an at-risk model? The answer to that question often defines the urgency with which you should think about post-acute care. In an ACO or a bundled payment model, you will face direct risk for post-acute behavior, and inappropriate post-acute utilization imperils potential savings.

Another key question involves owned post-acute assets. If you do own assets, your organization may be able to manage post-acute use and quality more directly and more quickly. This advantage is available only if your assets are properly positioned and optimized to perform. Oftentimes, however, they are not. Absent direct ownership, you can still engage with PAC but the approach will need to be different. The time it takes you to affect change in post-acute provider behavior might be longer.

Finally, organizational timeline is important as well. For instance, you might be predominantly fee-for-service right now and plan on becoming an ACO in next 12 to 18 months, but you have no owned post-acute assets and no defined post-acute strategy. This is where a majority of hospitals or health systems currently sit, especially as they step into ACO thinking. In this situation, the time to start engaging with post-acute care is sooner rather than later. Why? Because you ideally want post-acute care to be as high performing as possible before the ACO starts. In the first year of an ACO, one of the biggest opportunities for savings is usually in post-acute care. It often can take a year (at the very least nine months) to start seeing change and quality improvement in community-based post-acute providers. If you start your post-acute strategy after the ACO is initiated or at the same time, you'll miss out on the first year of potential savings.

What Are the Pain Points?

Your second level of consideration around post-acute strategy encompasses specific issues to address via improved post-acute engagement. In effect, you should ask, "What are the pain points that need to be considered?" Some of the more common pain points you can address or accommodate by post-acute care:

- Quality or performance outcomes, like readmissions or Medicare spending per beneficiary
- Acute length-of-stay challenges
- Patient satisfaction or care experience
- Specific risk for post-acute performance (care outcomes or quality)
- Organizational growing pains
- Market competition

These pain points, in combination with knowing where you stand, will often point you to specific engagement efforts with post-acute care. These specifics can help inform or craft your strategy. For instance, you might often experience acute length-of-stay challenges with patients that have certain diagnoses or clinical conditions. These patients who exceed length-of-stay targets and cost you money might be manageable in a post-acute setting. But you can't simply start discharging such patients to post-acute care. The PAC providers aren't ready yet. You will need to engage with them first to understand how you can work together to address this particular issue.

Where Do I Need to Be?

Finally, post-acute care is always likely to play a role in where you seek to be in the future. You likely want to be more integrated with the local market via greater risk relationships or to become a true population health organization—just to name a few possibilities. Given that post-acute services usually align with a hospital stay, there will always be close connectivity. It is sometimes easier for you to leverage the relationships and opportunities that are closest and position them accordingly. By way of example, an acute/post-acute alignment strategy is one of the first steps in building toward a broader continuum of care and establishing a foundation for clinical integration and longitudinal care pathways. Both of these approaches will lead you to better outcomes and happier patients.

Key Approaches to Acute/Post-Acute Engagement and Collaboration

There are many potential approaches for you around post-acute engagement (figure 8.4), and every market and organization is unique. Within this range of possibilities, however, the most common and usually successful efforts are grouped into three broad approaches: joint venture and ownership models; joint operating committees, collaboratives, or workgroups; and high-value or preferred provider networks. Each of these

Status Quo	Joint Operating Arrangements	Narrow or Preferred Networks	Joint Ventures	Sole Ownership
• No change in current discharge behaviors or patient management practices • Hospital or system utilizes wide array of post-acute providers with no regard for quality or outcomes • No investment required • No control over provider performance but can control volume	• Basic workgroup or committee relationship • Usually focused on fixing a problem or improving a particular process: care pathways or read missions • Overcomes disconnects and builds collaboration • Very limited investment • Slight influence over post-acute participants; volume redirection common	• **Aligned network** • **Emphasizes quality management of patients in PAC via careful and rugged selection of participants, redesign of care, and ongoing engagement** • **Invites modest investment to develop and maintain network infrastructure** • **Offers significant influence over participants; consolidates volume**	• Shared ownership, commonly with a post-acute managing partner • Usually involves new construction or redevelopment • Emphasizes quality management via shared ownership model but offers multiple challenges • Significant capital investment • Strong influence over operating partner but often insufficient volume for total need	• Fully owned and operated asset of the hospital or system; usually on balance sheet • Self-management challenges are very common • Comprehensive control over asset but opportunities to use incorrectly • Significant investment to purchase or develop ($200k–450k per bed); or costly to maintain, given age

Increasing Level of Hospital Control = Increasing Investment/Capital

Networks have emerged as the preferred solution for many organizations, given limited investment for significant return

Figure 8.4. Range of options for acute and post-acute engagement and collaboration.

offers varying pros and cons, and the ideal option for your organization will vary based on your evolution, culture, and strategic intentions.

Joint Venture and Ownership Models

Joint venture or ownership relationships represent the most capital-intensive approach as they often require investment in a shared relationship or outright purchase or development of a post-acute offering. If you need to exert full operational and quality control over post-acute care, ownership is the ideal approach. A joint venture relationship with another organization offers less direct control over either but still provides greater opportunity to influence than other approaches (figure 8.5).

Ownership is often challenging for some organizations because the desire to invest in post-acute services is greatly outweighed by other strategic options, such as building greater physician presence or developing outpatient or retail medicine models. Hospital and health system direct ownership of post-acute care is also often challenged by operational issues given the difference in post-acute operating models and the inherent variation in different post-acute settings—home health, skilled nursing facilities, and inpatient rehabilitation each operates in a different way.

Joint venture relationships have emerged as the ideal alternative to direct ownership because you can share the capital costs associated with building or buying; but more importantly, you typically involve a partner with specific knowledge or expertise who can direct or support the operations. Joint ventures among acute and post-acute organizations

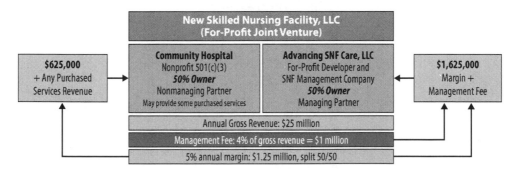

Figure 8.5. Example of a post-acute/acute joint venture arrangement.

have been more prevalent over the last decade than direct ownership, and they have typically encompassed hospitals partnering with a national or regional organization to develop skilled nursing and acute rehabilitation facilities. The capital commitment is shared, but the external organization manages the entity. As the hospital or ACO partner, you can influence quality and operations but share the risk for operational performance.

The downside of both ownership and joint venture is operational risk, although the degree is mitigated by full or partial ownership. Other approaches to acute/post-acute collaboration offer lessening degrees of operational or direct financial risk but can carry greater risk for quality performance and, in turn, impact financial performance down the road.

Joint Operating Committees, Collaboratives, or Workgroups

The concept of joint operating committees (JOCs), or collaboratives, has emerged in many markets across the country over the last several years. They represent a basic or starting framework for conversation among acute and post-acute organizations. The general structure is that of a chartered workgroup involving representatives from both sides that is convened to address a specific issue. Addressing readmissions or improving patient transfers are common topics for a JOC or a collaborative.

Given that improving communication among providers is always beneficial, JOCs and collaboratives are invariably a positive step forward. Despite longstanding relationships around discharging and admitting patients, the acute/post-acute interface is often very one-way—acute hospitals send and post-acute receives. The work is transactional, and given the nature of urgency associated with it, there is usually little time to work on the process itself. The JOC/collaborative framework creates a vantage point from which you can evaluate process and operational practice, and ideally tweak or improve it.

The ideal JOC or collaborative involves key leaders from both sides who are empowered to define and address the issue—such as a director of case management and staff along with a clinical lead and staff from post-acute. Executive sponsors on both sides are helpful to overcome roadblocks and garner broader organizational buy-in to potential remedies or solutions. Central to a successful JOC or collaborative is the charter document. The charter should clearly define the members and their related expectations around participation and engagement, the scope of work or problem to be covered, the anticipated outcome, logistics around meetings and scheduling, and so on. Absent a charter, the JOC or collaborative can quickly lose focus, wander outside of scope, and inevitably fail through lack of discipline.

The upside for you around JOCs or collaboratives is that they involve almost no financial commitment (beyond staff time) and, if managed correctly, can achieve desired results. The downside is that they are often very tactical, focusing on one or two issues, and their ability to leverage larger strategic, operational, and behavioral change is limited. Some organizations have managed to string together four or five JOCs, addressing various areas of concern of interest, but that approach either quickly breaks down under its own weight or gives way to a strategic approach around a post-acute network.

High-Value or Preferred Provider Networks

Perhaps the most dominant form of acute/post-acute engagement to have taken center stage in the last five years is the development of "high-value" or "preferred provider" networks. This network model typically offers you considerable opportunity to influence quality and utilization of post-acute care by consolidating discharges into a smaller, specifically defined pool of providers. While patients always retain choice and can choose any post-acute provider for their care, the inherent alignment associated with a network and the emphasis on quality and connection is appealing for many patients.

The network model is generally similar across most organizations (figure 8.6). A sponsoring entity—a hospital or an ACO—evaluates its local market for quality-oriented community-based post-acute providers. You then select potential participants via an evaluation process. This process typically involves publicly available quality data (often via CMS or other sources). The process assesses claims data and other informa-

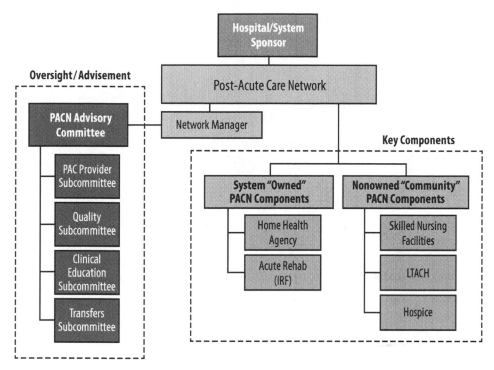

Figure 8.6. Preferred post-acute care network (PACN) structure.

tion that might be specifically requested of the potential provider pool. Once identified, post-acute organizations are engaged via some type of agreement or contract that defines expectations of participation.

The upside of networks for you is the ability to refine its relationship with a select group. As a result, the span of control is narrowed. The focus then is specifically on quality and utilization—two of the biggest drivers of post-acute cost. You'll find the costs associated with developing a network are far less expensive than a joint venture or ownership approach. In addition, your ability to extend relationships across a larger geography is greatly enhanced. This is particularly important because patients are typically inclined to choose post-acute options that are geographically convenient to them or a family member.

Governance and management of networks, however, are key to their success. You can't simply pick a group of providers and anoint them as preferred. To garner any measure of success, you must dedicate resources to manage the network daily, monitor quality and performance, and work with network members around quality improvement. A governance model must engage specific facets of the hospital or ACO that interact with post-acute care, such as case management, clinical leadership, emergency department, and the post-acute providers themselves. Through the governance structure and management, you can create specific workgroups or subcommittees to address a range of network development tasks. The likely tasks are redesigning transitions, advancing post-acute clinical skill, evolving palliative care approaches, and so on. Post-acute care providers are typically eager to engage in this work with the ACO. The work itself is defined as an expectation of participation but it also strengthens the post-acute care organization's relationship with you (upon whom they are potentially dependent). Importantly, it also inevitably improves their overall market position.

Considering Owned Post-Acute Care Assets

It's possible that you may own post-acute assets or have a small, self-contained continuum. For you these assets may have played a critical role in addressing particular challenges, such as acute length-of-stay throughput or addressing hard-to-place patients. In many instances, however, these PAC offerings are an afterthought when it comes to strategic thinking. As you think about the ACO and face increased pressure around cost and quality, your owned PAC assets should play an important frontline role in your PAC strategy, and they need to have a seat at your strategy table.

Optimizing for Performance

If you're considering integrating owned post-acute assets into either broader strategic thinking or a specific post-acute engagement approach—like a network—you need to be mindful of a few potential bumps that sometimes occur.

First of all, post-acute assets owned by a hospital or health system are often deployed and operated in ways that are different from their community-based cousins. Hospital-based or hospital-owned skilled nursing units sometimes serve as a setting for patients that represent acute length-of-stay challenges or are difficult to place elsewhere. As a result, the patient population in these units becomes highly diverse and often does not discharge quickly elsewhere. Expecting this type of unit to transform overnight (or within a short time frame) to an operation that rehabilitates and transitions patients quickly to meet a desired performance or quality target is usually a pretty big challenge. They will take time to change. By way of another example, hospital-owned home health agencies often do not have the same capacity or operational behaviors as proprietary operators. As a result, hospital case management staff is inclined to choose the faster, more responsive option. In many instances, the preference among case management staff is any agency other than the hospital-owned one.

Preferences among hospital staff for certain post-acute providers represent a second, and very real, bump in the road. You may want to believe that your staff will always choose their sibling option when it comes to post-hospital care, but the reality is often something very different. The very nature of "tribal knowledge" about options drives many of the decisions around post-hospital care. Discharge planners, case managers, and other staff involved in transitioning patients operate under daily pressure to "free up beds" and move patients through the hospital. As a result, those providers who are often most willing to take a patient are those who will get the patient—regardless of quality, cost, or organizational alignment. When it comes to promoting post-acute engagement within your organization, you're likely to discover that internal staff is frequently the biggest barrier to change.

Third, given bumps one and two and a history of having been simply overlooked, many hospital-owned post-acute assets simply don't perform at levels of operational or financial performance that align with their community-based competitors or their respective payment or reimbursement systems. This is not true of every single organization. Some hospitals and health systems do operate high-performing, high-quality post-acute programs—but they are in the minority. Given this preponderance, you should be prepared to ask very specific and introspective questions about the quality and capability of your owned post-acute assets. Operational evaluation or optimization may be an important step along the journey.

Why Owned Assets Often Aren't Enough

Beyond the operational and capability considerations, you also need to consider additional questions: Are my post-acute assets the right ones to have or do they have the capacity I will need? For most organizations, the answer is usually no. You may own an inpatient or acute rehabilitation unit, but you lack a home health agency. You may operate a hospital-based skilled nursing unit, but it only offers 18 beds. If we recall, 4 out of 10 Medicare patients end up in post-acute care, and a relatively similar number of Medicare Advantage patients go to PAC as well. If you pause for a moment and think about how many patients that might really be, your own internal capacity may be quickly overwhelmed. That quickly begs more questions: What's your approach to engagement with nonowned post-acute providers? Does it mean a network or a joint venture or some kind of collaborative effort?

Another consideration around the viability of owned assets is the often cultural or historical issues raised earlier. Can organization perceptions around how a post-acute asset has been deployed historically shift fast enough to address the new or emerging need? For some organizations, shifting cultural perceptions and behavior will require both an interim and long-term alternative—likely external providers.

Tactical Engagement with Post-Acute Care

As you start thinking about direct engagement and partnering with post-acute care organizations, an important—and somewhat relevant—proverb should come to mind: "physician, heal thyself." Many of the issues that challenge post-acute partnering grow from acute hospital behaviors and historical patterns. As such, you should take a good look at yourself as a first step in the process.

Historical Use

Rather than jumping right into post-acute provider quality data, you must also consider historical use of post-acute care and practices around discharge planning and referral to post-acute care. You should profile your discharge data to identify those post-acute providers receiving the bulk of historical referrals. This helps to identify both the scope and depth of post-acute distribution. In situations where patients are sent to multiple providers, your desire should be to consolidate post-acute use and improve span of control. In some instances, where scope of use is already narrow, the high-volume providers should potentially represent the key partners for consideration.

Case Management and Discharge Planning

In most instances, case managers and discharge planners are often a driving force for post-acute referral. As such, many will have established referral patterns—and sometimes those patterns are not aligned with highest quality providers.

You should begin by connecting with inpatient case management to get an idea of how the process works currently. The case or care management program is essential to ensure that services are coordinated across the continuum to allow smooth transitions at the appropriate levels as well as to guarantee a quality patient experience.

Seeking out their opinions and experiences with providers will further define the nature of existing provider relationships but also serves as a good barometer in how much work will be required to change case manager and discharge planner behavior around post-acute partnerships.

Connecting to Strategy

Finally, the evaluation of internal use should relate to your strategic considerations. What is driving the need for improved post-acute relationships? Is it in response to specific clinical conditions like joint replacement or cardiac procedures? Or does the focus relate to a desire to reduce acute length-of-stay or impact readmission performance? Understanding these specific issues is central to partnering efforts with post-acute providers and should ideally inform approaches to clinical integration and quality improvement efforts.

Overcoming Tribal Knowledge

If you're seeking better engagement with post-acute care, overcoming historical practices, perceptions, and misunderstandings is often one of the biggest hurdles. The array of "tribal knowledge" that exists in hospitals about post-acute care is often a guiding force in where patients go, how they get there, and who is involved in the process.

To that end, it's important to outline and know key steps in the patient progression of care in the hospital. Identifying specifics like what actions around discharge occur immediately upon admission to the hospital and what tasks are performed within 72, 48, and 24 hours of discharge can assist with performance improvement measures.

- How and when is the patient assessed for likelihood of readmission? Is the patient flagged in some manner to advise the post-acute provider of this higher risk?
- Is there some type of screening or evaluation that points to the ideal site of post-acute care based on patient status?
- How are post-acute options presented to patients and family members? Are recommendations made or implied about options, and who does that?
- Who is accountable for clear handoff and communication with the post-acute-based clinicians?

Evaluating issues around these questions, as well as many others, often reveal wide variation among hospital staff. Such inconsistencies can reveal potential barriers when it comes to a more formal post-acute partnering effort.

Picking Post-Acute Partners

You should think strategically about which post-acute providers you want to partner with or include in a network. When looking at potential partners, it's important to understand the gaps between the current and desired landscapes in order to create the infrastructure necessary to sustain a high-performing post-acute care network.

The Importance of Data

Available data on local post-acute providers offer a foundation to design an effective acute/post-acute care continuum. This continuum can improve linkages between the care settings and help inform who, where, what, and how these processes will be carried out for each patient. While macro trends have been documented on post-acute care variation for utilization, costs, and patient outcomes, providers will have to dig deeper to truly understand what's happening at a local level.

The Basics

Starting with the basics, you should take the opportunity to learn about the capacity and capabilities of all the post-acute care providers in the communities they serve, stratifying for details such as the type of post-acute care setting (i.e., skilled nursing facility or inpatient rehabilitation hospital), ownership (nonprofit vs. privately owned), and capacity (i.e., beds available or underutilized).

Having a sense of clinical leadership or existing relationships is also important. You should evaluate available quality and clinical measures, such as CMS five-star quality ratings, 30-day readmission rates, average length of stay or utilization, and patient and family satisfaction rates.

This data can typically be accessed via public domains, should shed light on the performance trajectory of local facilities, and serve to identify high-level challenges, such as widespread readmission issues or utilization. More detailed data, however, will be required when working through a selection process with potential partners to glean a more accurate view of the top performers.

Getting Deeper

If detailed claims data is available (either via participation in one of the alternative payment models or another source), you should conduct a thorough analysis of these data points. The interaction of various measures can be particularly telling. For instance, a post-acute provider with a shorter post-acute length of stay may be desirable, but if its readmission rate outweighs the cost associated with a slightly longer length of stay, it quickly becomes less appealing.

As you delve deeper into the variation that occurs post-acute, it's important to pay close attention to related clinical quality measures that inform a provider's track record and identify red flags that might challenge an effective partnership without significant process improvements.

Refining and Narrowing the Choices

After the deep dive on preliminary data, the next step is to begin the discussion with post-acute care providers within the local community to determine their level of interest in working with you. Selecting strategic partners requires a rigorous approach that should include not only comprehensive reviews of cost, quality, and market data but also an evaluation of post-acute provider capacity to meet your expectations.

A key goal early on is to garner enough information that will ultimately streamline the process to identify the right post-acute partners in the community. A best practice for many hospitals is to conduct a request for information (RFI) process to gather a wide range of data about the post-acute providers. Then you can start to winnow down the pool of potentially qualified applicants. RFIs should include extensive questions around size and capacity, ownership, facility or program leadership, staffing, clinical skills, quality measures, and other factors.

On-site visits of prospective post-acute participants are also beneficial when it comes to broadening the hospital or system's understanding of post-acute capacity and offerings. Via the on-site process, you can better equate outcomes and quality via interviews of senior leaders and key clinical staff and by touring a facility. During on-site visits, you and your team should consider the following questions:

- What is the physical environment—taking into account amenities and services, availability of private rooms, age of equipment, and general condition of the physical plant?
- What is the availability and response time of key ancillary services, such as pharmacy, specialized rehab, respiratory services, and lab and radiology?
- How does staff interact with patients and one another? Are there evident practices around customer service and patient experience of care?
- What is the post-acute provider's ability to accommodate the hospital's referral patterns (e.g., patient volume, time of day, patient type, average response time for referral requests, clinical complexity, discharging service lines)?

With RFI and site-visit results in hand, you are in a much better position to reconsider consumption and quality metrics and to ultimately segment the potential candidates into low- and high-performers. While selection criteria can vary among markets across the country, you should look for potential PAC providers that demonstrate or show a willingness to work toward markers of high-value care:

- Low readmission rates
- Average lengths of stay
- Top quartile performance for decreased fall risks and decreased infection rates
- Better than average patient-to-staff ratios
- High patient and family satisfaction scores
- Engagement in integration and care redesign

Selection and Preferred Provider Agreements

After culling through this baseline assessment work and data, you should be equipped with the right information to identify potential partners. These partners should be willing to share or align with your strategic post-acute needs or intentions. In addition, they should offer a culture that aligns with your organization's values around safety, quality, and patient-centeredness.

Preferred post-acute partners set themselves apart as top performers that can deliver the best quality and cost outcomes. They also successfully manage medically complex patients and commit to ongoing performance improvements. Leading candidates should, ideally, possess adequate capacity (i.e., beds, resources) that can meet service volume requirements; achieve suitable utilization targets and possess high-quality clinical services capabilities (or have the ability to develop them); and fulfill unique service needs in relation to the geographic distribution of the patient population. Overall, partners must be willing to agree upon overarching strategy and goals, adopt practice tools, and implement processes that standardize patient experience and promote quality outcomes.

Once partners have been identified and selected, new collaborative or preferred provider agreements will need to be developed. Post-acute and acute care providers will have to work together to create specific goals that improve quality and ultimately impact total cost of care. Most forward-looking post-acute organizations recognize that they can no longer operate as if they're in a silo. Many are eager to see themselves as an extension of the hospital or health system.

To that end, provider agreements must define expectations around collaboration, consistent communication, and data sharing. As relationships evolve and integration occurs, these value-based agreements will evolve to address risk-based payment and potential gain-sharing methodologies.

Building and Managing a Network: A Continuous Cycle of Plan, Do, Study, Act

As organizations build toward a potential network, it's important to determine roles and responsibilities internally to ensure hospital leaders and relevant stakeholders are fully aware of both your intent and expectation around post-acute engagement. There is a need to define who oversees leadership and management of the network and who has ownership and accountability for implementing, monitoring, and improving network operations. Many organizations have stepped into post-acute partnering without clearly thinking about how it will all get done.

Key Roles and Leadership

In the early stages of post-acute partnering and selection, it's often best that you develop some form of workgroup or committee to manage and inform the process. This group should ideally engage individuals across the hospital who are impacted by post-acute care and may play a role in the development process. At the very least, a workgroup should include both an administrative and a clinical lead. Additional individuals should represent care management, finance, quality, emergency department, information technology (IT), education, and communications. As the network evolves, these functional areas will be essential in both providing input to its development and supporting collaboration with post-acute providers.

With respect to senior leadership, a C-suite or comparable champion is critical as part of the network development process, which is likely to encounter challenges to historical thinking and practices. A C-suite champion who recognizes the importance of post-acute care will be the person to help overcome these challenges.

Network Management and Advisement

Building infrastructure to manage, monitor, and guide the network through development and operation represents a critical third step. The ACO must create an internal organizational structure for system resources that will support the network's reporting relationships, leadership champion, and ancillary areas such as IT, clinical education, and communications. A master working plan, documents, and tools must also evolve, including contracts, participating provider agreements, conditions of participation, and committee charters, just to name a few.

Because a post-acute network involves individuals and resources across a wide range of organizational areas and potential participating organizations, a committee structure that addresses supervision, oversight, and communication is also important. Network infrastructure should include some form of central or "coordinating" committee that encompasses members across all relevant disciplines. As with any infrastructure or governance effort, clear charters and expectations are important to the management process.

The top-level committee is supported by a series of subcommittees that can be specifically focused on clinical or operational areas. For instance, subcommittees might be established to address clinical education needs, IT collaboration, or care transition issues. These are aspects of the important clinical transformation work that is to follow once providers have been selected and agreed to participate.

Clinical Transformation

For many post-acute providers, meeting ACO expectations around improved patient outcomes, increased quality, and reduced costs will require investments of time and resources. These investments will aid in developing and enhancing their clinical skill sets and capacity. As a network developer, you can (and should) play a leading role in supporting this development process. ACO-sponsored clinical training and on-site clinician deployment serve as key elements in the dynamic transformation of acute/post-acute care.

Addressing Post-Acute Clinical Capacity and Skill Development

Appropriate staffing and skill sets are crucial to delivering quality post-acute care and typically make the difference between a quick recovery and a relapse or complication. The post-acute clinical team must be ready to admit patients in the post-acute facility on a 24/7 basis. Around-the-clock staffing of registered nurses has emerged as a minimum expectation in skilled nursing facilities to ensure patient safety, improve management of patient conditions, and prevent rehospitalization. The window of time to initiate care for a home health agency has been shrinking from 72 hours to as little as 24 hours in some organizations. Post-acute clinicians should employ evidence-based practices—such as the Interventions to Reduce Acute Care Transfers (INTER-ACT) quality improvement program—to assess changes in status, communicate with other clinicians, and make appropriate determinations around care.

The provider selection and accompanying site-visit process often reveals the clinical deficits and challenges that will need to be addressed. Post-acute organizations may have specific issues with treatment and management of certain conditions—such as congestive heart failure or chronic obstructive pulmonary disease—or they might be challenged with patient transitions or medical management. Addressing these issues via team-based approaches to analysis and redesign, using the subcommittee approach, has often proven an ideal solution. Engaging directly with post-acute providers to redesign and train in a collaborative approach helps both sides understand one another better. The result is better outcomes—and better care—for the patient.

Utilizing Options and Waivers

The various CMS ACO initiatives offer some specific waivers and options for both incenting and optimizing PAC use, especially with a group of preferred providers. Of most interest is often the "three-day skilled nursing facility stay" rule. For a Medicare patient to qualify for a Medicare-covered stay in an SNF, CMS typically requires that a patient spend at least three days in an acute hospital prior to the SNF stay. This can be a barrier for many patients who spend only one to two days in the hospital, are only ever at the hospital for an observation stay, or are diverted from an emergency department. The waiver allows for selected

SNF providers to receive Medicare payment for these patients (who did not stay for three preceding days).

This rule has considerable application for many ACOs (who must specifically apply to CMS to use it), and it carries certain requirements that must be met. For instance, the ACO must specifically inform CMS about which SNFs they will partner with and utilize an affiliate agreement for each facility. Partnering SNFs must also have an overall CMS quality rating of three stars or higher. Given these requirements, waivers are usually best considered for use as a result of a network development process, rather than via an arbitrary selection of market SNFs. It's also important to note that using this waiver will require certain clinical and performance capabilities to address patients with shorter hospital stays or those who have been diverted from an emergency department because they may be more clinically or medically complex. Again, a select group of vetted and capable providers (ideally arranged via a network) is an essential foundation.

Many ACOs have found success utilizing the three-day waiver, but it's important to understand that its use is very market specific. An ACO should well understand its SNF partners as part of its consideration and deployment. The application of other waivers—such as the post-discharge home visit, telemedicine use, and opportunities for gain-sharing with PAC—should be evaluated as part of a PAC network maturation process.

Driving Quality in Post-Acute Care

Given the investment of time and resources dedicated to partnering with post-acute care sites, you must be equally interested in ensuring the long-term success of the PAC providers. While there are subtle differences from one organization to the next, a post-acute partnering effort, such as a network, should emerge as an essential component of any future-looking strategy. To that end, it's essential that you develop a framework that seeks quality outcomes and ongoing dialog among all parties around process and quality improvement.

The role of outcome and quality metrics is central to post-acute engagement as the health system should desire to partner with providers that can address both quality and costs. Metrics additionally serve to distinguish the selected providers from others and to provide the basis by which participants will either remain in or be removed from the network.

Developing Measures

Creating the process for developing quality measures or metrics should involve both the ACO and the post-acute care organizations. The process should emphasize a core set of desired measures that address the challenges identified early in the network development, such as readmissions, rates of community discharge, post-acute utilization, patient satisfaction, and so on. Some may parallel the ACO's broader quality measures; others might be specific to a particular post-acute setting. Both parties need to agree on defined metrics to monitor outcomes, improvement, and quality. For example, utilization targets should be discussed by condition and also assessed based on needs of each patient. This is an evolutionary process and will require incremental development to set up preferred partners for success.

Once measures are defined and agreed upon, you should employ an initial data-gathering period (e.g., six to nine months) to establish baseline performance among the post-acute partners before promulgating specific performance expectations to all participants.

Reporting Data and Quality Improvement

While most forward-looking post-acute organizations deploy electronic health records, many do not yet have the infrastructure in place to share data electronically within health IT systems. As such, partners must agree and establish quality reporting time frames and data submission practices to ensure consistency among network members and establish the bases for comparisons. Outcome data should be shared openly among participants via the desired meeting process for discussion and feedback. The data should also inform potential opportunities for performance improvement. By way of example, trends around the specific clinical condition of complex wounds should inform the clinical education and training around improving wound management.

Key Ingredients for Success

While there are many avenues of opportunity around quality and savings within an ACO framework, an important part of your success will hinge on how you approach post-acute care and engage with post-acute care providers. Success with PAC organizations is never a by-product of chance, and if left alone, PAC providers will invariably always seek to optimize their payment, which means higher costs for you. To that end, there are several considerations and ingredients for success that you might consider as part of your PAC planning:

- Recognize the opportunity and need for an aligned engagement strategy for PAC, ideally a network but potentially one of the other approaches discussed herein.
- Find the right leadership in your organization, both executive and operational—this is critical.
- Evaluate current resources dedicated to care/case management, discharge planning, and acute/post-acute relationships and understand how they've operated historically and what future changes will be required.
- Understand that you may potentially need new resources or solutions—there are likely to be new roles required and investments in technology or professional guidance.
- Create a system for identifying the right partners—there is ample quality data and PAC provider data now available to inform selection.
- Develop quality metrics to collect and share. It's essential to use data to guide long-term management of a network and as a basis for improved performance over time.
- Engage with partners to drive clinical transformation and integration; you must work directly with PAC providers to get them to both buy in and change. You can't set arbitrary expectations and magically expect results.

NINE

Data Analytics

Making a Choice

SHAWN GRIFFIN

This is a difficult chapter as it won't answer the question you are asking. Data analytics is what most accountable care organizations at the outset want and trip over. Which analytics firm to pick is a challenge because the companies all say they do everything and do it well when, in fact, most do not. You need to come to grips with this dilemma. Shawn uses a judicious approach to explain this area and avoids any specific company recommendations.

Introduction

The analysis of data in managing populations serves to promote or create information to improve the care delivered by your providers. Data analytics can be the basis for a unified "shared platform of truth" that will drive provider behaviors and should not be mistaken for a goal itself. Analytics should communicate progress toward goals as a network matures. To be successful, analytics must strike an acceptable balance between timeliness and completeness. Accept that it will never be "perfect" to your providers, and show a willingness to discuss the known compromises required to produce a useful report. The compromises are whether it is timely or complete enough to use.

Many argue that internal analytics capabilities are a differentiator among groups that correlate with financial success. Admittedly, financial success can be supported by advanced data capabilities, but it by no means guarantees success. This chapter will focus on the evolution of analytics within a network from the initial role of communicating and/or repackaging information ("post office role") to the creation of new insights from combining cost, quality, clinical, demographic, cultural, and other data sources that fit the current buzzword of "big data."

There are several frameworks for the spectrum of analytics promoted by numerous organizations, and I will not endorse a particular one, except to note that the practical range from descriptive to predictive analytics with genomic data inclusion probably covers the playing field today. Much like the development of electronic medical record (EMR) capabilities of the past decade, scales exist that mark stages of development, but most organizations will recognize that due to distinctive characteristics of organizations, the same organization may have advanced capabilities in certain areas, or with certain sets of providers, but fail to deliver even the most rudimentary capabilities in other areas. This variation is often reflective of the data and cultural "kingdoms" that exist among providers and payers—sometimes due to lack of interoperability and sometimes due to lack of interest in sharing with possible rivals. This variability of information must also be seen within the culture of the organization since the exact same report could be viewed as incredibly useful by highlighting care gaps or as a "shaming" exercise within another network. As with most things in health care, your mileage may vary.

Vendors Provide Tools, Not Culture Change

There is no shortage of vendors who have products designed to assist in the area of analytics. Vendors have arisen from both within health care and moving into health care from other service areas. The newness of deeper analytics in health care (and the growth of population management by providers) has created a "gold rush" of start-ups and companies with limited health care understanding who are marketing services and tools that have not been tested across a variety of real-world providers. Some products have little to offer beyond a web domain and mock-ups in a presentation. They may not even know that HIPAA (the Health Insurance Portability and Accountability Act of 1996) *is not* a female hippopotamus.

The vendor area demonstrates the classic hype/marketing buzz conundrum seen with most technologies. All vendors should be viewed with caution. Significant questioning should be initiated to verify what they offer has shown capability with real data in the real health care environment and at a successful scale. It is not unusual to hear a vendor say, "Once you give us all your data, we can do great things with it," and gloss over those thorny problems of data acquisition and understanding the strategies to "fill in" the gaps that have always existed in health care data from multiple sources.

In my decades of assessing software, vendors, and emerging technologies, my personal preference has always been to speak with other users similar to my organization, use industry assessments such as KLAS (www.klasresearch.com), and insist on contracts that provide both limited financial exposure and input in ongoing development if a product is successful. Remember that a tool may work well in an isolated community with a single integrated delivery network on a common EMR but will rarely behave as robustly, for example, in a metro area with three major systems and 50% independent offices.

Importance of Contracting Well

The most important limiting factor in the ability of a team to create useful analytics is the raw information that is available for use—the classic "garbage in/garbage out" problem. For outside-sourced information, the quality and timeliness is often defined during the initial contracting process. Be sure that the operational teams that will spin data into insights will be adequately represented in the discussions *before* the contract is signed. Align your incentives in the contract with both the transparency and timeliness of the information flow to your providers' teams. It is very difficult to produce monthly reports highlighting gaps in care when the payer cannot provide the information except for every six months *and* it is three months delayed. Providers can manage reports one month old so long as that information is communicated as part of the distribution process. In our accountable care organization (ACO), our primary care physicians specifically asked for monthly reports on contract metrics highlighting gaps among their patients as a requirement for improving those metrics before the end of the contract period. Your data sources should be updated monthly, but due to small sample sizes in monthly information, performance reports should be based on at least six months of data to avoid wild swings in performance due to variation in small samples.

Payers also have limits within their systems regarding both financial and quality reporting. Traditionally, financial information has been timelier for payers as their systems serve as the ultimate financial ledger while clinical quality has been challenging for them to define without the full clinical record. Make sure that your contracts align incentives for both the payer and the providers to be successful.

Many organizations will avoid risk-based contracts until they have had at least one year of experience with the data from a payer. That will allow experience with the data cadence and the ability to understand what can be known with the information provided by the payer. It also provides a year to foster the operational relationship between support staff from the payer and your analytics groups, provider offices, and care managers. New payer data sets can reasonably be expected to take over six months to "stabilize" as a source for provider reporting. Also, any contractually required blinding of outside information (typically contracted amounts or provider identifiers), and the downstream effects that has, must be assessed for the degree that it impairs analysis or management.

The most important *financial* amount needed in claims is the paid amount. That amount serves as the basis for all calculations of member spending and physician-level reports of cost efficiency, typically reported as per member per month or per year. All information shared between payers and providers also must include appropriate restriction on the usage of the data. This data usage restriction is of greatest concern when a payer contracts with an organization that is also a payer—typically a provider-sponsored health plan. In these situations, the sharing of outside payer data with an inside payer organization would be both a legal and ethical violation.

Another area of sensitivity for the payers around sharing data with providers is when a provider organization is using analytics tools supplied by a competing payer organization, such as Aetna claims being given to a provider that uses Optum (part of UnitedHealth Group) for analytics. These potential conflicts have encouraged many providers to build their own analytics teams and departments using internal resources, but data protection and usage clarity should be part of all contract discussions.

Attribution

Attribution is assigning responsibility for a person or event to a specific individual or group. Within population or ACO analytics, this typically refers to the provider or providers *financially responsible* for the care of a member of an insured group. It is important that everyone involved understand that there may be a difference between "clinically" controlling the care and being financially accountable. There is no universally accepted model for ideal attribution due to the varied nature of care relationships and the reasonable exceptions to any one model. Most models for financial attribution will either assign responsibility to a primary care physician (PCP) based on a care relationship already established or through the selection of a provider during the insurance enrollment process. Required selection of a PCP was common during previous times of managed care and is becoming more common in tighter-controlled networks with some insurance plans.

Differences in attribution are also determining factors for participation in federal programs, such as the Medicare Shared Savings Program (MSSP). To oversimplify government regulations, Tracks 1 and 2 of the MSSP use preliminary prospective attribution based on services with final retrospective beneficiary assignment. Essentially, you get a list of members who probably will be yours, but you don't know for sure until the year is done. Therefore, your providers should treat every Medicare patient as though they might be in the program and not just focus quality and efficiency efforts on the members in your attribution file from Medicare. For Tracks 1+ and 3, the Centers for Medicare and Medicaid Services (CMS) uses prospective beneficiary assignment, which means you are approximately 98% sure who you should focus on. However, CMS removes beneficiaries that meet a limited set of exclusion criteria from each ACO's prospective assignment lists. This occurs on a quarterly basis throughout the performance year and annually at the end of each benchmark and performance year. The full details are found in about 30 pages of regulatory guidance available from CMS on the web.

Each contract should contain clear language about the methodology that will be used in the contract, and that definition should be acceptable to both parties. The contract should also include how attribution will be handled for persons that do not have a care relationship with any provider in the network.

One of the important clarifications needed in each contract is how to handle outreach to unattributed members. Some members will be concerned about the privacy of their medical information when contacted by a centralized resource, and the contract should be explicit that this outreach is permitted by the insurer for quality improvement efforts. This contract language should be echoed in the language used by the plans at member enrollment. This communication with members can also be important for HIPAA reasons and to avoid complaints when an unfamiliar person reaches out to a member to engage in supporting care.

In plans without a required selection of providers, there is often a large number of members who do not have a known provider relationship, and that population can derail quality improvement and efficiency efforts of the network. It is also very difficult to hold a provider accountable to either quality or financial targets influenced by a member they have never seen. Sometimes outreach must be performed at the network level to drive assignment of a member to an available provider. It is also useful for the benefit design in the product to encourage engagement with a PCP to facilitate care and attribution. This is particularly helpful when a change in payer leads to disruption in the members' usual care relationships with providers.

Evolution of Capabilities

In the beginning of the analytics journey, most networks (whether a clinically integrated network, an ACO, or an integrated delivery network) will begin with distribution of reports generated by a payer while the network develops in-house capabilities for more in-depth analytics. Development of analytics support will be dependent on talent availability and system resources. Some organizations start with borrowing or sharing resources from more mature parts of the organization, but that may be limited due to unique skills or the need to keep information domains separate.

At each stage of the development journey, the focus should be on producing operational tools that empower the network and are consistent with the strategic messaging from the network. Use your tools and teams to produce meaningful reports that show value and don't fall into the reporting trap of overwhelming information that paralyzes the providers. It is better to give a simple report that drives one focused effort than to produce a binder each week that is full of possible work but not one clear goal.

A generally safe place to start is to focus on contract-related metrics reports and educate your providers about their benchmarked performance compared to their network peers. Educate your providers on financial performance measures and show them the variation in performance among their peers. It may be best to have group meetings with blinded data slides to show the variation so they don't drill down to their own performance too quickly and miss the team aspects of performance that drive the overall contract success. Figure 9.1 represents an early example of the unblinded reports we shared with our providers at their regional meetings. These reports focused on contract metrics that drive overall cost and educated our providers regarding the main cost drivers and quality metrics in the population.

External Financial and Quality Reporting

For many groups, the first step in creating the shared truth of data is the distribution and/or reformatting of externally sourced information. This may include clinical or financial metric reports derived from submitted claims to the payer. This external information will usually be based on post-adjudicated claims reports that are frustratingly out of date and incomplete for providers. These reports can be useful at a high

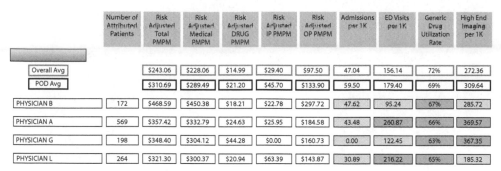

	Number of Attributed Patients	Risk Adjusted Total PMPM	Risk Adjusted Medical PMPM	Risk Adjusted DRUG PMPM	Risk Adjusted IP PMPM	Risk Adjusted OP PMPM	Admissions per 1K	ED Visits per 1K	Generic Drug Utilization Rate	High End Imaging per 1K
Overall Avg		$243.06	$228.06	$14.99	$29.40	$97.50	47.04	156.14	72%	272.36
POD Avg		$310.69	$289.49	$21.20	$45.70	$133.90	59.50	179.40	69%	309.64
PHYSICIAN B	172	$468.59	$450.38	$18.21	$22.78	$297.72	47.62	95.24	67%	285.72
PHYSICIAN A	569	$357.42	$332.79	$24.63	$25.95	$184.58	43.48	260.87	66%	369.57
PHYSICIAN G	198	$348.40	$304.12	$44.28	$0.00	$160.73	0.00	122.45	63%	367.35
PHYSICIAN L	264	$321.30	$300.37	$20.94	$63.39	$143.87	30.89	216.22	65%	185.32

Figure 9.1. Example of regional performance reporting for a group of primary care physicians. "Overall Avg" is the average performance on contract metrics across all providers in the system and the "POD Avg" is the average performance among this particular pod of providers grouped by region. Major drivers in spending included the risk adjusted spending total per member per month (PMPM), risk adjusted medical spending PMPM, risk adjusted drug spending PMPM, risk adjusted inpatient (IP) spending PMPM, and risk adjusted outpatient (OP) spending PMPM. Also counted were admissions per 1,000 attributed members (1K), emergency department (ED) visits per 1K, a generic drug utilization rate, and high-end imaging (i.e., CT scans and MRIs) per 1K.

level financially to demonstrate areas of cost that providers typically do not control within their clinical practice.

Population health will require that your providers understand that these previously "external" cost drivers can be the difference between achieving goals and incentives or falling short. These reports can also be used to highlight clinical or disease gaps, such as lower than expected rates on quality metrics that can be addressed by quality improvement programs at the network level and supported by outreach and EMR optimization at the clinic level. Most providers believe that any quality report should be supported by patient-level detail to allow closure of any known care gaps.

Payer Data Available to Providers

One of the newest areas of analytics for provider groups is payer-based analytics. This data set includes both attribution files and claims-sourced data. The "full claims" set provides the most complete financial picture for the calculation of total costs paid for care. Admittedly, claims do not provide the full clinical picture found in the EMR, but it still provides an invaluable insight into the full breadth of care given to a population.

Depending upon the benefit design and competitive geography, claims can highlight gaps in geography or capabilities of the network, leakage of services, and referral patterns. Leakage of services is often an area of emphasis for a network both for its implications on care being delivered outside the incentivized providers and the increased usage of in-network facilities to improve market share when appropriate. Due to delays in submission and processing of claims, the financial information is approximately 75%–85% complete for reports one month old, 88%–92% complete after two months, and 90%–95% complete after three. All reports and projects must recognize this aggregation rate when tracking over time to avoid underestimating most recent spend.

Integration and Influence of the Electronic Medical Record

Ideally clinical systems provide a comprehensive real-time view of care delivery. Care is often delivered by networks that exist on fragmented care platforms and that fail to achieve this ideal aggregation of relevant information. Many organizations have taken the approach of consolidating as many of their employed and aligned providers onto the dominant clinical platform of the funding organization. The dominant platform is often the inpatient facility or integrated delivery network. When caring for a population, I am not aware of a single large population that receives all clinical care on an integrated single platform, although some come close.

Every network has a long-term financial and clinical strategy for aggregating as much clinical information as reasonably possible into a longitudinal clinical record to improve care. In this environment, many vendors have added capabilities to their core EMR systems to serve as an organizational core system for analytics. True interoperability among EMR systems and portability of data would most likely displace many organizations from this restriction for analytics tools. Until that day occurs, the EMR platform is often the de facto data warehouse. This has created many interesting challenges due to the introduction of non-traditional information into the EMR-centric data framework.

As we discussed earlier, claims are not in real time or meant to be a complete record. This means that they are in some ways supplemental to the clinical record and introduce a number of new challenges in integration. Claims can be significantly time-delayed, not as detailed, and as they were for many years, not held to the same stringent rules that govern the clinical record. But the reality is that claims data, at least initially, will be the most complete and readily available source of some important data since clinical data has been harder to unify across systems.

Some payers also adopted rules for claims that make no sense in a clinical environment, such as Medicare Advantage requiring yearly documentation of chronic conditions that are clinically know to be permanent. There is also variability in the specificity of information in a claim (notably worse in some coding systems) than anyone would tolerate in a medical record.

For many years the purpose of the information on claims was to get a charge paid, not to document the subtle clinical difference important in delivering high-quality care. From a practical standpoint, claims information must be viewed with some suspicion before being given the same importance as information documented in the clinical record. I have seen claims that show pregnancy complications in an elderly man and prostate cancer in a ten-year-old girl. This data "pollution" has driven organizations to develop algorithms that give differing weight to various data sources and reflect the reliability of both the location of care and even the individual office based on their history of accuracy. Each data source should be assessed for accuracy when used for analytics. Processes should be created to improve any gaps in documentation in both the clinical and the claims records to provide the best and most complete information for analytics. Despite these gaps, claims traditionally serve as the "final say" in contract performance on both quality and financial outcomes.

Risk Scoring

The ability of an organization to document the variation in illness burden in a population should have an influence on the cost expected for their care. This is the concept of risk scoring. All analytics (especially when used for individual physician performance reporting) should include risk adjustment based on the documentation supplied by the provider. This is important because providers understand that sicker patients tend to be more expensive in a population.

When comparing the performance of providers, it is a familiar reflex for the provider with the higher cost population to say, "My patients are sicker." By accurately documenting the illness burden for a member, the expected cost will be adjusted to take that into consideration. This documentation provides the best apples-to-apples comparison among providers. If a physician is spending more on the care of a population on a risk-adjusted basis, there are only two options. Either the patients are more expensive than they should be (and the provider is responsible for that) or the patients' conditions contributing to the cost are not well documented (and the provider is responsible for that, too). Unfortunately, many providers were not previously educated on how to accurately document that risk in both the clinical record and the claims information to get "credit" for that condition burden. As contracts have evolved to hold physicians more accountable for the cost and quality of the care they deliver, more organizations have adopted documentation and coding improvement programs among providers to improve this data submission and, therefore, improve their reimbursement.

Summary

Remember that we are not talking about which data analytics firm you should hire. You will have to arrive at that conclusion the old fashion way—talk to other ACOs that have used vendors. Who did they like and why, and what did the vendor produce for them? Lastly, you may have to resort to trial and error in your own shop. What we can provide is some general guidance on the approach you should take to reach the conclusions you are after.

Data analytics for managing populations is a rapidly expanding area of focus for many organizations as they develop the capabilities to manage growing risk in contracting and improve the efficiency and quality of the care they provide. Like many transformative moments, this requires new people, new processes, and new technologies to be successful. Your ideal organization can build on current capabilities to begin educating your providers to the new language and realities of risk while expanding for future needs.

Most organizations will utilize new partners to develop platforms for data aggregation and provide the unified data environment to empower new activities, such as care management outside the traditional hospital and across aligned provider offices, ultimately moving into the post-acute world and the community. Integrating your provider organization early in the contract negotiations and viewing your contracts as a "portfolio of risk relationships" will be key in achieving contracts that support the consistent delivery of care and do not result in increasing burden on already-stressed providers.

It will bring into focus the subtleties of attribution and risk scoring and their importance on the accountability of providers to be both highly quality-driven and highly efficient. New data sets will be available (and required) to understand the broad scope of care locations and to show everyone who contributes to the process and who doesn't.

It will require new incentives to facilitate decreasing "waste" and to upset dynamics that have guided medical relationships. The wise organization will recognize that there is no one panacea, but instead a maturity curve of both culture and tools that must be linked to create a dynamic team that thrives in these uncertain times. No vendor or toolset will overcome an organization that cannot tolerate greater transparency and dependency on working together for the good of the community.

TEN

Impact of Coding and Documentation on Risk Scores

GLEN CHAMPLIN AND JOHN PITSIKOULIS

Accurate and specific coding will capture the correct acuity of your attributed populations. Hence your accountable care organization's historical benchmark will be adjusted by a risk score that is commensurate with the acuity of the population you are managing. Maintaining accurate coding and documentation also does not allow your risk scores to drop on continuously assigned beneficiaries. This supports better opportunity to generate shared savings for your organization and the Centers for Medicare and Medicaid Services. Glen and John emphasize the importance of a diagnosis being backed up by proper documentation and carefully enumerate the risk score components and their impact on the final risk score.

Coding and clinical documentation has become a new form of currency in Medicare. Risk scoring or a risk adjustment factor is now a performance metric in every Medicare value-based payment (VBP) model and is driven by a clinician's level of documentation specificity and coding accuracy to appropriately capture the true clinical severity of the patient population.

Coding and documentation will now also play a role in the reputational impact of your physicians via the Medicare Physician Compare star-rating website. Accurate coding and documentation also impacts revenue cycle management, denial management, and the transparency of the clinical data that your provider organizations want to utilize for risk stratification, predictive modeling, and care coordination across the continuum. Efforts in these areas can be more effective if the data being utilized to support them is as accurate and robust as possible.

The financial impact of risk adjustment in each Medicare VBP program is different based on your program design. In Medicare Advantage, where the impact is the most profound, it is used to adjust capitation payments to reflect what your potential prospective claims cost may be. In the Medicare Shared Savings Program (MSSP), it is used to normalize the benchmark target. But in all cases, this performance metric is used to adjust program financial outcomes. Based on the acuity of a population, risk adjustment helps your accountable care organization (ACO) account for the future potential expenditures of the beneficiaries attributed to your provider organization. In doing so, the intent of the Centers for Medicare and Medicaid Services (CMS) is to level the playing field. Risk score should advantage your provider organizations with populations that have a higher acuity than the average Medicare population. The new MSSP rule announced early in 2019 now provides an opportunity for ACOs to raise risk scores through accurate coding to adjust risk scores. This makes risk scoring an even more important performance metric for success in the new MSSP than in the previous version of the program. CMS added this upward risk score adjustment component to the new rule so that ACOs would not be disadvantaged on the basis that acuity generally rises as Medicare patient populations age.

The methodology for calculating the risk score is consistent with the various prospective payment systems developed by Medicare over the past 35 years. Under these methodologies, each case is categorized into a unit of payment based on patient demographics, diagnoses, and procedures, if applicable.

A similar methodology is used for assigning risk scores that are based on patient demographics and the health status of the population. Certain diagnosis codes for active and chronic conditions are designated as hierarchal condition codes (HCCs). Each HCC diagnosis is assigned a weighted risk adjustment factor reflective of predicted increased resource use. The HCC diagnoses are used in calculating the patient risk scores and adjusting providers' payments based on the complexity of the patient's health.

The risk adjustment factor of an attributed population in CMS VBP programs is determined prospectively by the amount of ICD-10 diagnosis codes retrospectively submitted via claims to CMS. It is important to note Medicare refines the HCC list of diagnosis codes on an annual basis to reflect changes in the conditions that impact the health status and cost to treat the population. HCCs are the coefficient factors used to adjust the baseline risk score that each attributed beneficiary receives. HCCs are also based on age, sex, and demographic status, such as being dual eligible. The risk score is then utilized in financial calculations pertinent, again, to the particular CMS VBP program design. Figure 10.1 illustrates an example of the impact of coding accuracy and specificity on risk score and capitation payments for an individual Medicare Advantage enrollee.

In this example, the additional HCC factors impact the overall risk score. The impact on the capitation payment is substantial and acts as an initial view into the substantive impact of risk score on overall VBP program performance. A critical component to the CMS risk score methodology is that conditions must be recoded year over year to

HCC/RAF Score Impact Case Study – Patient Level

Condition	ICD-10 Code	Relative Factor Score (health risk)	Demographic Score (85 y/o F)	RAW Risk Score	Total Payment ($800 community rate) x RAF Score
Type 2 diabetes mellitus without complications	E11.9	.104	.537	.641	$512.80
Urinary tract infection of specified site	N39.0	0.0	Not mapped to an HCC model category		

Condition	ICD-10 Code	Relative Factor Score (health risk)	Demographic Score (85 y/o F)	RAW Risk Score	Total Payment ($800 community rate) x RAF Score
Type 2 diabetes mellitus with diabetic nephropathy	E11.21	.318	.537		
Urinary tract infection of specified site	N.39.0	0.0	Not mapped to an HCC model category		
Major depressive disorder, recurrent, mild	F33.0	.395		2.315	$1,852
Status post below right knee amputation	Z89.511	.588			
Chronic systolic (congestive) heart failure	150.22	.323			
		.154	Interaction: congestive heart failure and diabetes group		

Figure 10.1. Medicare Advantage coding and documentation impact at the patient level on risk adjustment factor scores. Courtesy of Premier Inc.

maintain the previously established risk score unless a condition is no longer present and should not be coded. CMS designed the program in this way to support that all patients have an encounter and that care is delivered. Table 10.1 is a partial list of the ICD-10-CM codes (there are over 9,500) that are included in the 2019 CMS-HCC Risk Adjustment Model (Version 23).

While accurate coding is critical for capturing the severity of illness of the patient, documentation is at the core of every patient encounter. For clinical documentation to be meaningful it must be accurate, timely, and reflective of the clinical status that is translated into coded data. The coded data goes beyond reimbursement; it is translated into quality reporting, physician report cards, public health data, disease tracking, and trending.

Most importantly, good documentation is central to good clinical practice, and providers must document clearly, concisely, and at the highest degree of specificity. However, lack of documentation requirements, indifferences, poor habits, or a combination of these results in provider documentation deficiencies. Documentation specificity, in conjunction with the regulatory requirements, results in a complexity that requires education and training.

For example, documenting "LUL infiltrate" is poor documentation if the provider is treating left upper lobe pneumonia. "Will rehydrate patient" is poor documentation if the provider is treating dehydration. In both examples, the provider must document the diagnosis being treated—the coding guidelines prohibit the assignment of codes without the clear documentation of the diagnosis established.

For the purposes of this book, let us focus more specifically on the impact of risk score to the Medicare Shared Savings Program. In the MSSP, CMS develops predetermined cost targets and benchmarks as the barometer for determining qualification for bonus payments or penalties. CMS uses past performance to set a baseline for measuring future performance. Accurate risk adjustment plays a very important role in the evaluation of an ACO's performance.

In the new MSSP model, Medicare develops a benchmark that it will use during the five-year MSSP performance period. The initial

ICD-10-CM Codes[a]	HCC Category Description	HCC	Disease Hierarchy
B20, B97.35, Z21	HIV/AIDS	1	
A02.1, A20.7, A22.7, A26.7, A32.7, A39.2–A39.4, A40.–, A41.–, A42.7, A48.3, A54.86, B00.7, B37.7, P36.–, R57.1, R57.8, R65.1–, R65.2–, T81.12XA	Septicemia, Sepsis, Systemic Inflammatory Response Syndrome/ Shock	2	
A07.2, A31.0, A31.2, B25.–, B37.1, B37.7, B37.81, B44.0–B44.7, B44.89, B44.9, B45.–, B46.–, B48.4, B48.8, B58.2, B58.3, B59	Opportunistic Infections	6	
C77.0–C77.2, C77.4–C77.8, C78.–, C79.00–C79.72, C79.89, C79.9, C7B.–, C80.0, C91.0–, C92.00–C92.02, C92.40–C92.A2, C93.0–, C94.00–C94.22, C94.40–C94.42, C95.0–	Metastatic Cancer and Acute Leukemia	8	9, 10, 11, 12
C15.–, C16.–, C17.–, C22.–, C23, C24.–, C25.–, C33, C34.–, C38.4, C45.–, C48.–, C90.00–C90.22, C92.10–C92.32, C92.9–, C92.Z–, C93.10–C93.92, C93.Z–, C94.30–C94.32, C94.80–C94.82	Lung and Other Severe Cancers	9	10, 11, 12
C40.–, C41.–, C46.–, C47.–, C49.–, C56.–, C57.00–C57.4, C58, C70.–, C71.–,C72.–, C74.–, C75.1–C75.3, C77.3, C77.9, C79.2, C79.81, C79.82, C81.–, C82.–, C83.–, C84.–, C85.–, C86.–, C88.2–C88.9, C90.3–, C91.–, C95.10–C95.92, C96.–	Lymphoma and Other Cancers	10	11, 12
C01, C02.–, C03.–, C04.–, C05.–, C06.–, C07, C08.–, C09.–, C10.–, C11.–, C12, C13.–, C14.–, C18.–, C19, C20, C21.–, C26.–, C30.–, C31.–, C32.–, C37, C38.0–C38.3, C38.8, C39.–, C51.–, C52, C53.–, C57.7–C57.9, C64.–, C65.–, C66.–, C67.–, C68.–	Colorectal, Bladder, and Other Cancers	11	12
C43.–, C4A.–, C50.–, C54.–, C55, C60.–, C61, C62.–, C63.–, C69.–, C73, C75.0, C75.4–C75.9, C76.–, C7A.–, C80.1, C80.2, D03.–, D18.02, D32.–, D33.–, D35.2–D35.4, D42.–, D43.–, D44.3–D44.7, D49.6, E34.0, Q85.–	Breast, Prostate, and Other Cancers and Tumors	12	
E08.0–, E08.1–, E08.641, E09.0–, E09.1–, E09.641, E10.1–, E10.641, 11.0–, E11.1–, E11.641, E13.0–, E13.1–, E13.641	Diabetes with Acute Complications	17	18, 19
E08.21–E08.638, E08.649–E08.8, E09.21–E09.638, E09.649–E09.8, E10.21–E10.638, E10.649–E10.8, E11.21–E11.638, E11.649–E11.8, E13.21–E13.638, E13.649–E13.8	Diabetes with Chronic Complications	18	19
E08.9, E09.9, E10.9, E11.9, E13.9, Z79.4	Diabetes without Complication	19	
E40, E41, E42, E43, E44.0, E44.1, E45, E46, E64.0, R64	Protein-Calorie Malnutrition	21	
E66.01, E66.2, Z68.41, Z68.42, Z68.43, Z68.44, Z68.45	Morbid Obesity	22	

ICD-10-CM Codes[a]	HCC Category Description	HCC	Disease Hierarchy
A39.1, C88.0, D84.1, D89.1, E03.5, E15, E20.0, E20.8, E20.9, E21.–, E22.–, E23.–, E24.–, E25.–, E26.–, E27.–, E31.–, E32.–, E34.4, E70.–, E71.–, E72.–, E74.00–E74.09, E74.20–E74.29, E74.4–E74.9, E75.21, E75.22, E75.240–E75.249, E75.3, E76.–, E77.–, E79.1–E79.9, E80.0–E80.3, E83.110, E85.–, E88.01, E88.4-, E88.89, E89.2, E89.3, E89.6, H49.811–H49.819, N25.1, N25.81	Other Significant Endocrine and Metabolic Disorders	23	
I85.–, K70.41, K71.11, K72.01–K72.91, K76.6, K76.7, K76.81	End-Stage Liver Disease	27	28, 29, 80
K70.30–K70.9, K74.3–K74.69	Cirrhosis of Liver	28	29
B18.–, K73.–, K75.4	Chronic Hepatitis	29	
A54.85, K25.1, K25.2, K25.5, K25.6, K26.1, K26.2, K26.5, K26.6, K27.1, K27.2, K27.5, K27.6, K28.1, K28.2, K28.5, K28.6, K50.012, K50.112, K50.812, K50.912, K51.012, K51.212, K51.312, K51.412, K51.512, K51.812, K51.912, K56.–, K59.31, K63.1, K65.–, K67, K68.12, K68.19	Intestinal Obstruction/ Perforation	33	
K86.0, K86.1	Chronic Pancreatitis	34	
K50.–, K51.–	Inflammatory Bowel Disease	35	
A01.04, A01.05, A02.23, A02.24, A39.83, A39.84, A50.55, A54.4–, A66.6, A69.23, B06.82, B26.85, B42.82, M00.–, M01.–, M02.1–, M02.8–, M02.9–, M46.2–, M46.3–, M72.6, M86.–, M87.–, M89.6–, M90.5–	Bone/Joint/Muscle Infections/Necrosis	39	
L40.5–, M02.3–, M04.–, M05.–, M06.–, M08.–, M12.0–, M30.–, M31.0–M31.7, M32.–, M33.–, M34.–, M35.00–M35.3, M35.5, M35.8, M35.9, M36.0, M36.8, M45.–, M46.00–M46.1, M46.50–M46.99, M48.8X–, M49.8–	Rheumatoid Arthritis and Inflammatory Connective Tissue Disease	40	
D46.–, D46.A, D46.B, D46.C, D46.Z, D47.4, D57.0–, D57.1, D57.2–, D57.4–, D57.8–, D59.–, D60.–, D61.0–, D61.1, D61.2, D61.3, D61.82, D61.9, D66, D67, D75.81	Severe Hematological Disorders	46	48
D61.8–, D70.–, D71, D72.0, D76.–, D80.–, D81.1–D81.7, D81.89, D81.9, D82.–, D83.–, D84.0, D84.8, D84.9, D89.3, D89.8–, D89.9	Disorders of Immunity	47	

Source: Amerigroup. *CMS-HCC Risk Adjustment Model (V23): ICD-10-CM to CMS-HCC Crosswalk.* Washington, DC: Amerigroup; 2018. https://providers.amerigroup.com/Documents/ALL_CARE_CMSHCCRAModel.pdf. Accessed November 5, 2019.

Note: "There are over 9,500 ICD-10-CM diagnosis codes that map to one or more of the 83 HCC codes included in the 2019 CMS-HCC Risk Adjustment Model (Version 23). A code can map to more than one HCC as ICD-10-CM contains combination codes (i.e., one code can represent two diagnoses or a diagnosis with a complication).... The CMS-HCC Model [also] incorporates disease hierarchies, in which payment will only be associated with the most severe manifestation of a disease.... The table includes the HCC category descriptions, along with the HCC code and associated disease hierarchy. The model and mappings ... are subject to change with updates to the ICD-10-CM codes."

[a]The diagnosis codes listed with a dash indicate an expanded code category of additional codes that are available based on disease specificity.

benchmark is risk-adjusted using the CMS-HCC model that is based on the risk score developed for the attributed patient population from benchmark year three data. When setting these targets, CMS uses data on the historic reimbursement it has made to providers to identify what the historic cost of the attributed population has been. Then CMS determines the projected cost by applying trend factors and a risk adjustment factor (RAF) score to the historic costs for the attributed Medicare population. The cost baseline is developed using the historic data for the previous three years of claims reimbursements with a differential weighting applied to each of the three years. The RAF score is developed based on the diagnostic coding and documentation submitted by the provider's claims to Medicare in baseline year three. The calculated HCCs identify the complexity and acuity of the patient population. These scores are aggregated across ACO attribution subpopulations (e.g., aged dual, aged nondual) into average group risk scores, which are then used in the benchmark adjustment or calculation.

The case mix index, which is a relative value assigned to the diagnosis-related group of patients in the inpatient environment, is used in determining the allocation of resources to care for and/or treat the patients in the group. The RAF score is the equivalent relative value assigned to the whole patient population to determine the allocation of resources based on the beneficiaries' average HCC assignments.

Then each year over the five-year performance period an interim benchmark calculation is performed to adjust the prospective benchmark for change in the prospective cost of your ACO's attributed population. This accounts for deaths, new attributees, and other factors in the establishment of the benchmark, such as inflation trends and the change in risk score.

Once the initially attributed MSSP population's risk score is established, these lives are called the "continuously assigned patient population." In the old MSSP rule, the risk score for patients in this population, once developed from benchmark baseline data, could not be adjusted upward over the life of the contract performance period, but it could be adjusted down. Downward adjustments would occur if a condition that generated an HCC was no longer present and therefore no longer available to code, or if codes previously submitted in claims that converted into HCCs were not again captured in subsequent claims submissions, then the loss of HCCs would create a downward adjustment in risk score for the individual patient. If enough of this loss in coding accuracy and specificity occurred across the patient population, a possible downward adjustment to the group risk score utilized in the interim benchmark calculations could occur. There was and is today no cap on the level of downward adjustment that can occur. A significant risk score reduction can seriously impact all Medicare VBP performance results, and historically it has proven to be very detrimental to the chance of producing shared savings for most ACO groups in the MSSP that have experienced a downward risk adjustment. ACOs must develop and deploy processes and education that insure that their health care providers are recapturing all relevant previous diagnoses and that these diagnoses are billed on every patient encounter every year.

Via the new rule, risk scores for the continuously assigned population can now go up if coding accuracy and specificity improves or if new conditions not previously coded arise and are captured. The increase is subject to the 3% cap in the interim benchmark calculations.

For newly assigned beneficiaries, an ACO's updated CMS-HCC prospective risk scores should take into account the changes in severity and case mix for these newly assigned patients. Newly assigned beneficiary risk scores are assessed, and if their average is different from the average HCC score of the ACO's original population, the benchmark is adjusted for this population. These beneficiaries would then convert to the continuously assigned category for future risk score calculations.

Since the HCC methodology is designated as a hierarchal condition code set, diagnosis lacking documentation specificity and inaccurate coding can result in the underreporting of accurate diagnostic codes, which is turn results in lost revenues. For ACOs that historically have not performed well at coding diagnoses, if they can drive performance improvement in accurately capturing the highest level of specificity for all diagnostic codes, then they should be able to improve their RAF score and cost benchmarks.

In most instances, newly assigned beneficiaries are individuals aging into Medicare. ACOs must stress the importance of identifying and engaging these patients to encourage encounters in the first year of attribution in which the provider, and in most cases a primary care provider, is diligent about capturing all diagnostic codes. This, along with recapturing all previously submitted codes on continuously assigned beneficiaries, creates the best opportunity to positively impact recalculation of the RAF score and adjustments to the benchmark during the interim performance period savings calculations.

As discussed, accurate health assessment of new and continuously assigned beneficiaries is critical for your organization's success within the Medicare Shared Savings Program. It is important for groups considering entry into the MSSP to evaluate the effectiveness of coding within their physician population. You can then understand in a directionally correct manner the impact current coding performance will have on the benchmark calculations performed by CMS. It may be prudent for some provider organizations to delay entry into the program. During the delay, they can improve coding accuracy and specificity to ensure that the RAF score of the potential MSSP-attributed patient population is more reflective of the actual acuity and complexity of their patient population as well as insure that the possibility of a downward risk adjustment is minimized.

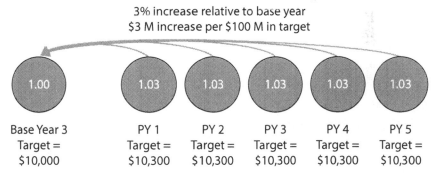

Figure 10.2. Potential impact of a maximum 3% upside but unlimited downside benchmark adjustment. This does not include the annual Office of the Actuary adjustment, national or regional trends, or regional adjustment caps. Courtesy of Premier Inc.

As previously stated, the new MSSP rule allows the benchmark to be adjusted using the full relative HCC risk score change, up to a 3% increase. This would provide some mild protection to ACOs that see a less healthy population in the performance year while allowing Medicare to retain savings if an ACO enrolls a healthier population. The final rule does not limit benchmark reductions for risk score changes—not adopting the proposed 3% floor on risk adjustment reductions—which would have effectively allowed ACOs to keep costs associated with a significantly healthier population. An example of the potential impact is highlighted in figure 10.2.

Historically, most clinicians have not seen the connection between accurate coding and documentation and financial success in population health management programs. They have seen this activity as an additional administrative burden that did not contribute to delivering better patient care or generate any additional reimbursement. As the evolution of VBP progresses, it will become ever more important for clinicians to excel in the area of coding and documentation. It will also become important for the organizations that support these clinicians to model the financial impact of risk scores on VBP programs. In so doing, organizations should provide financial evidence for why risk scores are such an important performance metric. Clinicians will then understand why accurate coding and documentation and the effort it requires are vital to driving performance assessment and improvement.

In conclusion, regardless of whether you are a group considering MSSP participation for the first time, continuing your current ACO strategy, or looking to change to a different payment model, the importance of a continuous commitment to HCC capture and RAF score accuracy cannot be stressed enough. No matter which way providers turn today or in the future, the implications of good performance in accurate coding and documentation and risk score capture are critical to the success of an ACO. The importance of this effort will only grow more consequential with time.

[ELEVEN]

Legal and Compliance Considerations

SETH EDWARDS

Medicare had to change certain health care laws in order to make accountable care activities legal and to permit each organization to operate as a group entity. Once legally formed, accountable care organizations (ACOs) must comply with the Centers for Medicare and Medicaid Services (CMS) recommendations in order to continue to be certified as an ACO and an integrated health care delivery organization. New rules and waivers enacted as a result of the 2018 CMS rule changes are discussed here.

Introduction

As we have discussed throughout this book so far, the world of health care is evolving, and the tactics and strategies for success in the value-based world of accountable care organizations differ from those necessary in a fee-for-service environment. This dynamic is also true as you analyze legal and compliance considerations for ACOs. This chapter will provide you with an overview of the changes occurring in this area of population health and how organizations are using the new rules to facilitate success.

The fee-for-service payment system utilized by the Centers for Medicare and Medicaid Services includes many rules designed to protect against fraud and abuse. As CMS and other payers continue to shift to value-based reimbursement models and require health care providers to accept more financial risk, the need for these payment rules will lessen. During the development of the Medicare ACO programs, CMS recognized this dynamic and worked with other parts of the administration, including the Federal Trade Commission and the Department of Justice, to create multiple waivers designed to allow enough flexibility for

ACOs to successfully manage an aligned population. CMS expects Medicare ACOs to comply with the new regulations by creating their own policies.

In addition to the fraud and abuse waivers, CMS has also started testing additional payment waivers, which are available to ACOs participating in two-sided risk models (i.e., the models where an ACO is at risk for both shared savings as well as shared losses). These waivers are designed to test adjustments to payment rules with a goal of facilitating achievement of the Triple Aim: lower cost, better outcomes, and better experience of care.

In order to create a model that can successfully leverage the waivers outlined, CMS has created numerous requirements that must be achieved in order for your ACO to qualify for participation in the program. These include organizational requirements, program integrity, data security, and public reporting. Monitoring compliance with these elements is critical for continued participation in alternative payment models.

As the ACO is being created and after it is approved, it is critical that each ACO write policies that

- outline the composition of the governing body,
- create an organizational chart,
- establish a conflict of interest policy,
- obtain physician acknowledgement of participation agreements,
- design and approve committee charters,
- develop business associates agreements,
- document and implement marketing plans,
- originate a website for public reporting of ACO processes and results, and
- initiate many other related procedures.

As a part of this approach, your ACO has many considerations that have legal and compliance ramifications.

Overview of Waivers

With financial risk shifting from CMS to ACOs, many of the rules associated with the fee-for-service system have become archaic. To address this dynamic and create an environment in which ACOs can operate and be successful, CMS has developed fraud and abuse and payment rule waivers. The fraud and abuse waivers are largely available to all Medicare ACOs, while the payment waivers are largely being tested with two-sided risk ACOs. In addition, CMS has, with a few exceptions, limited the applicability of the payment waivers to models that include prospective assignment of beneficiaries. This is necessary in order to ensure that the waiver is being applied appropriately to ACO-assigned beneficiaries.

Fraud and Abuse Waivers

CMS and the Office of Inspector General, in conjunction with other parts of the federal government, have made available five fraud and abuse waivers for Medicare ACOs. These waivers remove the application of the Stark law, the Anti-Kickback Statute, and the Civil Monetary Penalties Law.

Pre-participation waiver
The pre-participation waiver is available to ACOs planning to apply for a Medicare ACO model. It can be used for ACO-related start-up arrangements in anticipation of participating in a Medicare ACO model.

Participation waiver
The participation waiver is the continuation of the pre-participation waiver and applies to ACO-related arrangements that occur during the ACOs participation in the Medicare ACO model.

Shared savings distribution waiver
The shared savings waiver allows for the distribution and utilization of the shared savings payments earned as a part of the Medicare ACO

program, also appropriately known as the Medicare Shared Savings Program (MSSP).

Stark law compliance waiver
The Stark law compliance waiver removes the barrier imposed through the potential of anti-kickback and civil monetary penalty laws that implicate the Stark law within the Medicare ACO models.

Patient incentive waiver
The patient incentive waiver allows flexibility for medically related incentives to be offered by the ACO under the MSSP to encourage preventive care and compliance with treatment.

Payment Waivers

In addition to the fraud and abuse waivers and in conjunction with other related parts of the administration, Health and Human Services has made available multiple payment waivers (1).

Skilled nursing facility three-day rule waiver
The skilled nursing facility three-day rule waiver eliminates the requirement in fee-for-service Medicare that a beneficiary be admitted to the hospital first as an inpatient for no fewer than three consecutive days prior to being admitted to a skilled nursing facility (2).

Telehealth originating site waiver
In fee-for-service Medicare, telehealth service billing is largely limited to rural health professional services areas. This waiver eliminates the rural geographic originating site requirement and allows for the use of asynchronous telehealth services in the specialties of teledermatology and teleophthalmology (3).

Post-discharge home visit waiver
This waiver gives providers greater flexibility in billing evaluation and management services provided to beneficiaries after discharge. It eliminates the direct supervision requirements for incident to billing services (4).

Beneficiary incentive program waiver

Established under the Pathways to Success MSSP 2018 rule, this waiver allows ACOs to establish a beneficiary incentive program where the ACO can provide an incentive payment or certain in-kind gifts, not to exceed $20 for each qualifying services the beneficiary receives through the ACO (5).

As noted previously, each Medicare ACO model has specific waivers available for use. The figures here outline the applicability of the waivers for each ACO model under the current program (figure 11.1) and as evolved under the Pathways to Success structure (figure 11.2).

Compliance Requirements

As you will see, the applicability of the fraud and abuse waivers is extremely broad and may allow arrangements that are currently prohibited or present material risk to the Stark law, the Anti-Kickback Statute, and Civil Monetary Penalties Law. The pre-participation, participation, and shared savings distribution waivers apply to the ACO, ACO participants, ACO provider/suppliers, and outside providers and suppliers who have a role in ACO activities. The waivers are also

Waivers	MSSP Track 1	MSSP Track 1+	MSSP Track 2	MSSP Track 3	Next Generation ACO
Fraud and Abuse					
Pre-participation waiver	X	X	X	X	X
Participation waiver	X	X	X	X	X
Shared savings, distribution waiver	X	X	X	X	X
Stark law compliance waiver	X	X	X	X	X
Patient incentive waiver	X	X	X	X	X
Payment					
Skilled nursing facility 3-day rule waiver		X		X	X
Telehealth originating site waiver					X
Post-discharge home visit waiver					X

Figure 11.1. Waivers available to Medicare Shared Savings Program (MSSP) ACO models.

Waivers	MSSP Track 1	MSSP Track 1+	MSSP Track 2	MSSP Track 3	Next Generation ACO
Fraud and Abuse					
Pre-participation waiver	X	X	X	X	X
Participation waiver	X	X	X	X	X
Shared savings distribution waiver	X	X	X	X	X
Stark law compliance waiver	X	X	X	X	X
Patient incentive waiver	X	X	X	X	X
Payment					
Skilled nursing facility 3-day rule waiver		X		X	X
Telehealth waiver		X		X	X
Post-discharge home visit waiver				X	X
Beneficiary incentive program waiver				X	

Figure 11.2. Waivers available to Medicare Shared Savings Program (MSSP) ACO models under Pathways to Success and the Bipartisan Budget Act of 2018.

considered self-executing, and ACOs do not need to receive approval from a federal agency. This differs from the payment waivers, which require an application and formal approval prior to utilization.

Use of these waivers requires that the ACO is participating in the Medicare ACO program and meets the requirements for the program related to governance, leadership, and management. For the fraud and abuse waivers, the ACO's governing body must have made a bona fide determination that the arrangement is reasonably related to the goals and purpose of the Medicare ACO program (1). CMS has not provided specific requirements to outline how an ACO makes a determination of an activity or arrangement being reasonably related to the purposes of the ACO, but the ACO must "articulate clearly the bases for the determination." The waiver identifies the purposes of the program as one or more of the following items:

- Promoting accountability for the quality, cost, and overall care for a Medicare patient population
- Managing and coordinating care for Medicare fee-for-service beneficiaries through a Medicare ACO model

- Encouraging investment in infrastructure and redesigned care processes for high quality and efficient services delivery for patients (4)

In addition to the requirements already outlined, each ACO is required to publically report their utilization of each waiver. The majority of ACOs place this information on their public website. CMS does not expect the disclosure requirement to be overly challenging or onerous, and it does not require the disclosure of economic terms in order to meet the requirement. The disclosure must occur within 60 days of the beginning of the arrangement.

Summary

As payment and delivery models continue to transition risk to providers, the archaic rules associated with the fee-for-services system will become less necessary. As a part of that transition, CMS has begun to make available fraud and abuse and payment rule waivers to ACOs. These waivers provide for much greater ability for your ACO to function successfully and to engage with beneficiaries to reduce costs, improve outcomes, and enhance patient experience. Clear understanding and evaluation of the waivers, expectations for compliance, and potential pros and cons for each is critical for your ACO's success as a compliant, legal organization.

REFERENCES

1. Buck C, Healy P. Medicare ACO participation waiver of fraud and abuse laws: how it works and why ACOs should use it. *AHLA Connections*. 2014;18(12):20–23.

2. Three-day inpatient hospital stay requirement for care in a skilled nursing facility [FAQ sheet]. Baltimore, MD: Center for Medicare and Medicaid Innovation; 2018. https://innovation.cms.gov/Files/x/nextgenaco-threedaysnfwaiver.pdf. Accessed April 10, 2018.

3. Next Generation ACO model: telehealth expansion waiver frequently asked questions [FAQ sheet]. Baltimore, MD: Center for Medicare and Medicaid Innovation; January 2018. https://innovation.cms.gov/Files/x/nextgenaco -telehealthwaiver.pdf. Accessed June 17, 2018.

4. Medicare program; final waivers in connection with the Shared Savings Program; interim final rule. *Fed. Regist.* 2011;76(212):67992-68010. To be codified

at 42 CFR. https://www.federalregister.gov/documents/2011/11/02/2011-27460 /medicare-program-final-waivers-in-connection-with-the-shared-savings-program. Accessed June 17, 2018.

5. Centers for Medicare and Medicaid Services. *Medicare Shared Shavings Program: Beneficiary Incentive Program Guidance.* Baltimore, MD: CMS; 2019. https://www.cms.gov/Medicare/Medicare-Fee-for-Service-Payment/sharedsavings program/Downloads/BIP-guidance.pdf. Accessed April 10, 2018.

TWELVE

Employee Health Management and the Role of an Accountable Care Organization

JEREMY MATHIS

Efficient accountable care organizations are often asked to manage the employee health plans of the practices with which they are associated. As pointed out by Jeremy, this is a golden opportunity for employers to not only reduce their costs of health care, but also to improve the culture of the organization and the engagement of the employee in the process. Employee health plans should produce healthier employees who will have better care and disease management and be more productive. Costs can be reduced for both the employer and the employee. This is a key chapter for the business community.

Introduction

Understanding the "why" and "how" of employee health plan management requires a keen focus on your health care system and the role an accountable care organization (ACO) could play in your employees' health.

- Why are America's businesses, not just health care systems, investing in ACO strategies and tactics for their employees?
- How are health systems addressing employee health?
- Which tactics are producing the greatest impact and why?
- How are employee health programs being integrated with other population health initiatives?

Answers to these questions can be gleaned from the industry research, experience, and learnings of the Population Health Management Collaborative's Employee Health Plan Cohort at Premier Inc. The cohort has been operating for more than six years and includes approximately 50 health systems, all actively managing self-funded employee health plans. Here is what we've learned.

The "Why"—Why Health Systems and Other Employers Should Invest in Accountable Care Strategies for Their Employee Health Plans

The US Congressional Budget Office recently reported that private spending (e.g., payments by private health insurers, consumer out-of-pocket spending, and other miscellaneous expenses) accounts for approximately 35% or $1.6 trillion of total health care spending in the United States (1). In 2019 private health spending grew by 6% (2), and industry experts are projecting even larger growth in 2020. This rate far exceeds the consumer price index increase in the US in 2019 (3). Additionally, employer health spending as a percentage of wages has increased considerably over the past decade (1), impacting the growth of employee compensation.

Because of these trends, employers are shifting a greater portion of the premium to their employees to soften their organizations' burden associated with rising costs. This strategy can only be tolerated for a short while. Employer patience is dwindling. To correct the cost trend, they now realize the need to take action on their own. They cannot wait any longer on providers, insurance carriers, brokers, and third-party administrators for a new approach.

Warren Buffett identified the locus of this issue when he recently stated that "medical costs are the tapeworm of American economic competitiveness" (4). We are seeing employers with similar perspectives step outside of traditional models. In order to lower costs, employers are taking more control in hopes of driving greater health plan performance. The most notable example in recent news is the new collaboration of Amazon, Berkshire Hathaway, and JP Morgan. In 2018, they announced that they are forming a joint venture with the purpose of providing low-cost and high-quality health care to their employees. Since introducing the organization, they have hired a senior executive and named the organization Haven. The industry is anxiously waiting to learn more about Haven's strategic initiatives and focus, as well as the impact they will produce.

The issue of rising premiums spans all industries and is the leading reason why organizations, likely including your own, invest in employee health programs. The National Business Group on Health and Optum recently conducted a study focused on understanding why employers offer health and wellness programs and whether their reasons go beyond health care cost savings. The study found that the primary reasons for investing in health and wellness programs are reducing employee health risk, reducing employee health care costs, and improving employee productivity (5). All three can be tied to decreasing health plan costs and premiums.

In addition to cost reduction opportunities, we must also note that there are significant strategic and cultural reasons to invest in employee health and wellness. In fact, the previously discussed survey also found that 91% of all employers offer health and wellness programs to their employees for reasons beyond medical cost savings. Does yours?

Let's take a closer look at each of these incentives that contribute to a compelling argument for why employers, including your organization, should invest in employee health.

Financial

Most employee health insurance plans within the health care system and other large organizations are self-funded rather than fully insured, and there are many operational differences between the two. Most pertinent to our focus is who assumes the financial risk. Under a fully insured plan, an insurance company assumes the financial risk for the employer on a yearly basis. If your organization's employee health plan is fully insured, there is a fixed premium that it is responsible for paying each year. However, its insurer would have the ability to increase premiums each year while providing limited visibility into the factors that warrant an increase. A positive aspect of a fully insured plan is that with a fixed premium for each year, your organization would have a greater ability to confidently budget each year's health care expenses and reduce risks associated with sharp spending increases or high cost claimants.

Contrary to fully insured plans, many employers, particularly large employers, have self-funded health plans for their employees. If your organization's health plan is self-funded, it has likely obtained some form of stop-loss insurance to protect against significant spikes in spending, but in general it would assume total financial risk for its employees' health care costs outside of that protection. It also would likely pay a fixed cost to a third-party administrator to manage plan administration functions, such as claims processing. However, the largest portion of its cost under a self-funded model would be variable and based on its employees' claims. This structure, paired with effective management of care and developing a workforce that includes educated consumers of care, can lead to significant expense reductions to improve your organization's bottom line.

In addition to directly impacting the health care dollar, when designed appropriately, employee health programs can positively impact employee productivity, performance, satisfaction, and retention and decrease sick days within your organization. The Health Enhancement Research Organization recently reported that a range of 85%–97% of organizational leaders believe that a person's health significantly influences their performance and productivity (6). All these factors combined can lead to significant labor-related cost savings. Additionally for health systems, we must also consider how provider health translates to performance and ultimately to patient safety and quality outcomes.

Cultural

In conducting research for this chapter, I interviewed three large regional health care organizations to better understand why they invest in improving the health and well-being of their employees. Each organization shared that reducing cost is equally important as improving employee well-being and cultural alignment. To elaborate on this, let's consider an organization's mission statement, which is typically created to help define and communicate their purpose. If you do a quick internet search on your local health systems' mission statements or review your own organization's, you will likely find mention of improving the health, wellness, or satisfaction of the community, environment, or service area they operate in. For these systems to deliver on their mission, they must improve these factors as a whole for their own employee and dependent population, which typically make up a considerable portion of the health system's community. If they are not doing so, they are, in a sense, failing to deliver on their mission.

Employee health programs can also significantly improve employee engagement. A recent Gallup poll found that approximately 30% of employees working for large businesses feel engaged with their organization (7). This low level of engagement typically leads to a less than optimal alignment between employees and the organization's desired culture. However, if designed correctly, employee health programs can improve employee engagement and satisfaction. As you design your health program, select programs that can truly impact quality of life for your employees. Consider initiatives that reduce stress, improve morale, and bring people together. Improving quality of life and the work environment for your employees will typically lead to greater organizational engagement, retention, and alignment with your organization's culture.

Strategic

As I previously introduced, employers are facing the imperative of having to reduce the cost of care for their employees, which is likely true for your organization as well. However, patience with traditional cost containment tactics has expired because these efforts have produced minimal improvements. As a result, many particularly large non–health care provider organizations have begun testing innovative solutions to move upstream, closer to the initiation of patient care. More specifically, they are pursuing direct-to-employer agreements with health care provider organizations that exclude the insurer or payer. These new models typically consist of high-performing clinically integrated networks (CINs) or accountable care organizations as part of their health plan design to focus on managing total cost of care or specific episodes of care.

Direct-to-employer models are proliferating rapidly across the country and are expected to continue multiplying. PwC's Health Research Institute recently reported that 23% of employers are actively considering direct-to-employer agreements, and 34% are actively considering the inclusion of a performance-based network (e.g., an ACO or CIN) in their plan design (2). A few examples of these models include Adventist Health with Whole Foods, Henry Ford Health System with General Motors, AdventHealth with Disney, and national Centers of Excellence with Walmart, Boeing, Lowe's, and others for certain episodes of care.

As these models continue to grow, employers and insurers will pursue provider partners with established, performance-based networks that have a proven ability to decrease cost and improve quality and patient experience. To win these opportunities, you will be required to support the effectiveness of the capabilities within your organization by pointing to past performance results. In other words, employers will want to see evidence demonstrating how your ACO or CIN has produced cost savings and high-quality outcomes for a specific patient population before agreeing to trust your network with its own employee population. Therefore, you should consider your own employees as a testing ground for population health improvement. It is a strategic opportunity to demonstrate your organization's capabilities to other employer suiters.

By demonstrating positive employee health plan results, you may also be able to negotiate more favorable value-based terms with your payer partners—most specifically related to the delegation of services from the payer, or per-member-per-month payments from the payer, to your organization to support care delivery infrastructure and services. Positive results can be leveraged in negotiations to demonstrate your organization's capabilities and support certain requests that would benefit the patient and your ACO or CIN's ability to effectively delivery care.

The "How"—How Health Systems Should Address Employee Health Plan Management and Integrate and Optimize the Use of Clinically Integrated Networks or Accountable Care Organizations

Employers use several accountable care tactics and strategies to impact the performance of their employee health plans. However, in most cases, employee health programs are not comprehensive. Programs are often implemented in an order that does not optimize the program's impact and return on investment. Figure 12.1 provides the six key components of effective employee health plan management and the sequence in which they should be implemented or prioritized within your organization to maximize results.

Let's explore key characteristics for each of these capabilities, including implementation timing and integration with your ACOs or CINs.

Data Analysis and Reporting

Do not fly blind! Many organizations eagerly develop an employee health program without precisely understanding what they want to accomplish or what their employees' needs are. Arbitrarily designing your strategy can lead to wasted resources and minimal progress. That is why data analysis and reporting is the first step and the foundational building block for managing your employee health plan. Start with the basics:

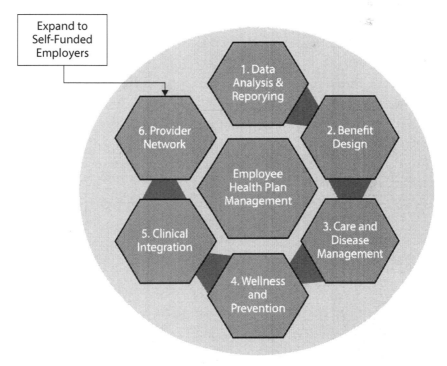

Figure 12.1. Employee health plan management: components and implementation sequence.

- Study your employees' environment.
- Review available socioeconomic data.
- Solicit input from your employees.
- Utilize your third-party administrator (TPA) to identify key areas of opportunity.

This information will inform your strategy and the resources that you will need to develop an effective program.

Your analyses will not only inform your strategy but will also track your impact and show you how to evolve your program over time. It is vital to develop a reliable reporting and analytics system with recurring reports provided on a consistent cadence. In most cases, relying on your TPA for these reports will be required initially. Over time, however, the program should integrate with your ACO or CIN's analytics capabilities to internally produce reports that will supplement the information that your TPA provides. Some basic examples of metrics that your reports should include and trend over time are as follows:

- Population characteristics: monthly enrollment (employees and dependents), age and gender distribution
- Financial: per-member-per-month cost trend, monthly incurred and paid claims (total and by care setting—inpatient, outpatient, professional, ancillary, etc.)
- Utilization: emergency department visits per 1,000 members, inpatient admission per 1,000 members, cost trend by disease state (e.g., musculoskeletal, diabetes, circulatory)
- Clinical: common disease states, average population risk score
- Network utilization: in- and out-of-network utilization by care setting
- Risk stratification: categorization of the population based on health condition parameters set by your organization or TPA, for example

low risk: generally healthy, low-utilizer of care;
stable: also generally healthy, higher utilizers of care, some risk to become high cost and could benefit from care support;
at risk: relatively high utilizers of care, conditions are not yet severe, high likelihood of becoming high cost;

chronic/struggling: very high utilizers, high cost, and health
   conditions significantly impacting day-to-day function; or
complex: usually has multiple chronic conditions, severe acute
   episodes, extreme utilizers and high cost

If your TPA is unable to report on these metrics, consider changing TPAs. These reporting capabilities are reasonable, and the functionality required to produce this information should be standard for administrators. The role of your ACO or CIN related to this capability is to eventually produce analyses and reports independently that supplement the reports provided by the TPA. These reports can be integrated with analytics developed for other value-based populations. Often it is an arduous process to enable an ACO or CIN to produce analytics for a health system's employee population. Due to privacy concerns, a firewall must be established and approved by the organization's legal counsel. The firewall will ensure that patient-level data is only viewed and used by those that need it for clinical purposes.

Benefit Design

Health plan benefit design is a powerful tool that can have a significant impact on cost and utilization when used effectively. However, benefit design can also have determinantal effects on employee satisfaction, recruitment, and retention if not balanced appropriately. It is a continuous process that does not cease. Design changes are made each year based on the needs of the population. For this reason, benefit design is the second priority in the model (figure 12.1). Regardless of the maturity level of an organization's employee health program, analytics continue to expose key opportunities. Recognizing the opportunities, an organization can make tweaks to its health plan design to incentivize or disincentivize certain behaviors.

Some common benefit design strategies that you should consider to reduce cost and improve employee engagement and self-ownership of care include the following:

Offering a high-deductible option
Each year we survey the Employee Health Plan Cohort (EHPC) participants on key trends, areas of focus, and lessons learned, among several other topics. The most recent survey found that 53% of participants now offer a high-deductible health plan (HDHP) option to their employees. This percentage is expected to grow for the next several years. HDHPs are certainly capable of reducing employer cost in the short-term. In 2017, the average annual premium for family coverage was approximately $1,200 less for a HDHP than other models (8). However, there are concerns that patients will avoid care due to high out-of-pocket cost and that long-term cost will increase due to a decline in health. Another concern that is of particular interest to health systems, due to the threat of bad debt, is the patient's ability to pay their medical bills under a HDHP. In an effort to offset these potential cons, as an employer you should consider pairing HDHPs with a health savings account. In addition, you should include incentives to encourage patients to consistently participate in preventative care practices.

Incentivizing the promotion of healthy living and preventative care
The incentives that your organization selects should be specific to its employees' needs. However, it is common to promote preventative care by incentivizing the completion of an annual wellness visit or health risk assessment. Incentives for maintaining or improving key biometrics, such as body mass index or blood pressure, which are indicators of overall physical health, are also common. You should be creative with the incentives and willing to develop customized strategies. However, you must always be aware of and abide by the laws that regulate wellness incentives.

Disincentives for using high-cost care settings
People are creatures of habit that love convenience. They also have preconceived notions about where they'll receive the highest quality care available. As a result, they typically do not avoid unnecessary care at high-cost care settings, such the emergency department or specialist physicians' offices, which can be significant cost-drivers for employers. To address this issue as an employer, you should implement higher co-pays

and other disincentives for using high-cost care settings if appropriate, lower-cost care settings are reasonably accessible. You should also provide education to employees focused on how to be good consumers of health care. The education should include a review of how to appropriately use high-cost care settings, such as the emergency department.

In addition to these tactics, employers are also shifting more cost to their employees in the form of higher deductibles and co-pays and the responsibility to pay a greater portion of the premium. On average, employees are now paying 24% of the total premium (9). The aforementioned EHPC survey found that health systems are requiring their employees to cover a range of 10%–30% of the total premium. Many of the organizations that are on the higher end of this range reported that they are beginning to receive pushback from their employees and are concerned about job retention and decreased employee satisfaction. As noted earlier, it is important to be very strategic and cautious about your benefit design strategies. Design changes can produce unintended consequences if they are rejected or negatively received by your organization's employees.

Care and Disease Management

It is atypical for an employer to implement care and disease management (CM and DM) programs before wellness and prevention programs for their employees. Frequently organizations begin with wellness and prevention programs because they usually require fewer resources, are easier to establish, and require a smaller capital investment. On the other hand, care and disease management programs can require a large number of licensed clinical staff, are more complicated, and require more one-on-one time with patients. Studies analyzing the return on investment (ROI) produced by both models vary. However, CM and DM programs do tend to produce a more immediate impact and return. Therefore, if CM and DM are initiated prior to a wellness program, an ROI may be available more quickly to reinvest into employee health programs and support the wellness program.

As an ACO or CIN, your role is to ensure that existing CM and DM infrastructure and strategy are integrated with the CM and DM initiatives for the employee population. The EHPC survey found that 52% of employee health plans have no functional integration with their organization's other population health services and infrastructure. This represents a significant missed opportunity to capitalize on shared learnings and to maximize economies of scale.

In addition to ensuring alignment and integration between your ACO or CIN and the health system, you must also develop a plan for how they will coexist with the disease management services offered by your TPA partner. Too often internal programs do not communicate or coordinate with the TPA. The lack of coordination leads to duplication of services and calls to patients. It also leads to a lack of information-sharing between programs. Each organization's model may be unique, but regardless of the model, CM and DM services should be integrated and aligned internally and externally. In many cases, the ACO or CIN is the optimal hub for coordinating and providing overarching leadership for CM and DM.

Wellness and Prevention

Do wellness and prevention programs (a.k.a. wellness programs) produce an ROI? This question has been a hot topic of debate in recent years. I would argue that the answer is dependent on the design and execution of each individual program. There is, however, still significant research supporting the ability of effectively designed programs to lower health care costs, improve productivity, and promote healthy behaviors (10). As this debate continues, I want to acknowledge that wellness programs are not intended to immediately produce a financial ROI and use this opportunity to review the more intangible aspects that are considered by many to be the backbone of employee health plan management.

Building upon this, another key takeaway from my recent interviews with three large regional health care organizations is that without employee engagement and a supportive culture, an organization's employee health program is severely disadvantaged. As you develop and design your organization's programs, you should not only evaluate the financial return of your wellness programs, but also evaluate their impact on topics such as health awareness, healthy behaviors and lifestyles, and overall organizational culture.

Each organization's wellness program will be uniquely designed and based on its employees' needs, but there are some consistent steps that should be taken by all organizations when developing a program to help increase the likelihood of success.

Brand your program

Develop a brand, name, and clearly stated purpose that are actively communicated to your employees. Each employee should be able to recognize and associate with the organization's wellness program.

Engage leadership

Company culture starts from the top. Engage all levels of management early to gain their support and participation. Also, consider inviting an executive to publicly endorse and speak about how they are utilizing the wellness offerings.

Engage and collect feedback from staff

Collecting input from your colleagues to develop and structure your employee health program is vital. Consider developing wellness committees that represent each area of the company to select wellness initiatives and objectives.

Engage providers

Solicit provider input and participation in the planning and design process for your wellness program. Their insights and support can lead to more impactful offerings and improve their engagement and the frequency in which they refer patients to the wellness programs.

Assess your current culture as a baseline

A baseline cultural assessment should be used to track progress and identify gaps between the current state and the desired future state. These gaps or opportunities should be used to help inform the services provided by your wellness program.

Clinical Integration

The Federal Trade Commission and US Department of Justice, in the *Statements of Antitrust Enforcement Policy in Health Care*, define a CIN as "an active and ongoing program to evaluate and modify practice patterns by the network's physician participants and create a high degree of interdependence and cooperation among the physicians to control costs and ensure quality" (11). When developing a comprehensive employee health program, you should view your organization's program as a part of the patient's care team. In doing so, take steps to comply with this definition by ensuring that your employee health program is cooperating and engaging with your CIN's or ACO's participating providers to control costs and ensure quality.

This is a more advanced step in the framework (figure 12.1) because it requires engagement and alignment with outside entities across the care continuum. This step is always a significant challenge. To get started, consider engaging with primary care providers and ensuring that they are aligned with any third-party vendor that may be providing your organization with employee health services. As organizations begin introducing CIN and ACO narrow networks, the ability to integrate clinically becomes much more obtainable due to the alignment of incentives. However, prior to a narrow network, health systems should begin moving toward clinical integration by taking the following four steps:

1. Invite certain providers from all specialties to participate in the planning process for designing the organization's employee health program.
2. Provide education to providers and ensure that they are aware of the employee health programs that are available to their patients.
3. Ensure that providers are offering to enroll eligible patients into applicable employee health programs. Providers should be automatically notified when their patient is eligible, and the enrollment process should be quick and simple.
4. Implement a system for sharing employees' participation and progress, and notify the patient's primary care provider of their program results.

Provider Network

Selecting and introducing a narrow provider network as a tier within an organization's health plan is another large and challenging step. This step can generate significant resistance from employees. It is also challenging to design because you must ensure that you have adequate network coverage with high-performing primary care physicians and specialists. For these reasons, this is step six in the framework (figure 12.1).

The EHPC survey of health systems found that 41% of participants currently offer a narrow network plan option to their employees. This is significantly higher than the national average that the Kaiser Family Foundation reported to be just 8% nationally for all industries in September 2017 (12). This number is expected to grow but is a good illustration of the challenge with implementing narrow networks and the advantage that health systems have and should leverage.

The high level of uptake by health systems may be attributed to the tendency for health system employees to live in a more geographically manageable area as opposed to other organizations that may have employees located in several different sites across the country. Additionally, it is very important to health systems that their employees pursue care within their own provider networks. Therefore, narrow networks commonly consist of health systems' employed and affiliated providers, which are then used to mitigate out-of-network use.

The advantages of a well-designed narrow network are significant. They can foster team-based, highly coordinated care; hold providers accountable for outcomes; and funnel employees to providers that have a proven track record of delivering efficient and high-quality care. And ACOs and CINs present a perfect opportunity for a health system to integrate a narrow network into their employee health programs. Most of these networks of providers already track and measure their ability to deliver high-quality, low-cost care and have incentive/compensation structures in place to drive desired outcomes.

If using an ACO or CIN to get started, you should first ensure that the organization or network provides adequate coverage. For many ACOs and CINs, you will be required to patch network gaps with other independent providers. Once network adequacy has been ensured, the ACO or CIN should be integrated into the health system's plan design as the tier-one option. Incentives should be offered to encourage employees to select this tier, such as lower premiums, deductibles, and/or co-pays. Additionally, performance metrics and incentives should be agreed upon by the ACO or CIN to reward participating providers for positive outcomes.

Expand to Self-Funded Employers

Health systems that build out each of the six capabilities shown in figure 12.1 and produce positive results will have developed a compelling value proposition and model that can be packaged, customized, and sold to other employers.

If designed appropriately, direct-to-employer models should benefit the patient, employer, and provider organizations (i.e., the CIN, ACO, and larger health system). A well-designed program is intended to create benefits for each party (figure 12.2).

These models are proliferating across the country and present great potential for market share growth and retainment for health systems.

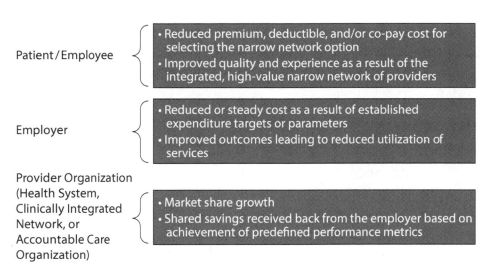

Figure 12.2. Contracting benefits for each player in well-designed direct-to-employer models of employee health plans.

Without being able to demonstrate a network's capabilities in its own employee population, health systems will be challenged to win direct-to-employer opportunities.

Summary and Key Ingredients for Success

Investing in the development of an employee health program is a financial, cultural, and strategic endeavor for employers. For health systems to optimize employee health plan performance, they must perfect a comprehensive program, including

- data analysis and reporting,
- informed and strategic benefit design,
- care and disease management,
- wellness and prevention,
- clinical integration with employed and affiliated providers, and ultimately
- the inclusion of a high-value narrow provider network tier within the health plan design.

Learning, developing, and optimizing these capabilities will better position organizations to effectively manage their own employees and organizational culture. They will also be strategically positioned for the future as employers move more rapidly toward more narrow, high-value networks and direct-to-employer agreements.

REFERENCES

1. Banthin J. *Health Care Spending Today and in the Future: Impact on Federal Deficits and Debt.* Presentation to a conference organized by the Center for Sustainable Health Spending. Washington DC: Congressional Budget Office; July 18, 2017. https://www.cbo.gov/system/files/115th-congress-2017-2018/presentation/52913-presentation.pdf. Accessed November 14, 2019.

2. PwC Health Research Institute. *Medical Cost Trend: Behind the Numbers 2019.* New York City, New York: PwC; June 2018. https://www.ehidc.org/sites/default/files/resources/files/hri-behind-the-numbers-2019.pdf. Accessed November 14, 2019.

3. Consumer price index summary [news release]. Bureau of Labor and Statistics website. https://www.bls.gov/news.release/cpi.nro.htm. Published May 2018. Updated October 10, 2019. Accessed November 14, 2019.

4. Sorkin AR. Forget taxes, Warren Buffett says. The real problem is health care. *New York Times*. May 8, 2017.

5. Marlo K, Serxner S. Beyond ROI: building employee health and wellness value of investment [white paper]. Eden Prairie, MN: Optum; 2015. https://www.optum.com/content/dam/optum/resources/whitePapers/Beyond_ROI_health-wellness-investment.pdf. Accessed November 14, 2019.

6. HERO Health, Productivity, and Performance Study Committee. *Exploring the Value Proposition for Workforce Health: Business Leader Attitudes about the Role of Health as a Driver of Productivity and Performance*. Edina, MN: Health Enhancement Research Organization (HERO); February 2015. https://hero-health.org/wp-content/uploads/2015/02/HPP-Business-Leader-Survey-Full-Report_FINAL.pdf. Accessed November 14, 2019.

7. Gallup. *State of the American Workplace*. Washington, DC: Gallup; 2017. https://www.gallup.com/workplace/238085/state-american-workplace-report-2017.aspx. Accessed November 14, 2019.

8. Rivera A. The pros and cons of high deductible health plans. *Business News Daily*. April 30, 2018. https://www.businessnewsdaily.com/10723-pros-cons-high-deductible-health-plan.html. Accessed November 14, 2019.

9. Willis Towers Watson. *High-Performance Insights—Best Practices in Health Care: 2017 22nd Annual Willis Towers Watson Best Practices in Health Care Employer Survey*. London, UK: Willis Towers Watson; 2017.

10. Black A. Five reasons employee wellness is worth the investment. *Health.gov Blog*. May 17, 2017. https://health.gov/news/blog/2017/05/five-reasons-employee-wellness-is-worth-the-investment. Accessed October 28, 2019.

11. US Department of Justice and the Federal Trade Commission. *Statements of Antitrust Enforcement Policy in Health Care*. Washington, DC: Federal Trade Commission; August 1996. https://www.ftc.gov/sites/default/files/attachments/competition-policy-guidance/statements_of_antitrust_enforcement_policy_in_health_care_august_1996.pdf. Accessed November 14, 2019.

12. Claxton G, Rae M, Long M, Damico A, Foster G, Whitmore H. *2017 Employer Health Benefits Survey*. Menlo Park, CA; Chicago, IL: Henry J. Kaiser Family Foundation and Health Research & Educational Trust; 2017.

THIRTEEN

The Role of Primary Care in the Future of Health Care

MOREY MENACKER

Most approved accountable care organizations (ACOs) are led by primary care providers (PCPs). "In the past," Dr. Morey Menacker writes, "PCPs have not had the same cachet as specialists." A PCP himself, Morey explains why PCPs, then, are the logical leaders of ACOs and what their obligations as leaders are. To be successful, the PCP should ensure the interests of the patient, improve care quality, minimize waste, and reduce costs.

Introduction: Evolution of the Primary Care Physician

One hundred years ago, the medical school graduate had limited choices of specialty. There was the surgeon, who worked in the hospital and mainly dealt with traumatic injuries; the diagnostician, who was a professor at the medical school and was asked to evaluate patients whose illnesses were not well recognized; and the family doctor, who saw patients in the office, made house calls, delivered babies, and managed a full spectrum of complaints.

As diagnostics and therapeutics developed, physicians migrated to concrete areas of specialization in order to develop and maintain expertise in a limited area of medical care. However, to this day, the overwhelming amount of care is devoted to treating the sick, not to maintaining health. The term "health care" is actually a misnomer, whether discussing the financing of services or the focus of providers. A more apt term would be "sick care."

In the 1980s, an attempt to standardize physician compensation resulted in the resource-based relative value scale, which was used to set fees for physician services. Procedural fees far exceeded diagnostic or consultative fees. This led to a migration of medical school graduates to procedural specialties. This change further eroded the role of the family doctor in patients' minds as well as the status of the profession. The internist, the pediatrician, and the obstetrician/gynecologist were replacing the family doctor. This further led to a fragmentation of care, with various specialists competing for different parts of each patient's body (and wallet).

The insurance industry's response to this explosion of costs was to create the health maintenance organization (HMO). If you were a primary care provider, you would have been designated as a "gatekeeper." Your role was to block the torrent of diagnostic testing and limiting cost. You were compensated based on the number of patients you controlled and not on the care you provided or the outcome of your treatment. Specialists were contracted with limits on their compensation yet were continued to be paid for volume only. Interestingly, most data suggest that outcomes slightly improved while utilization decreased. However, the public was dissatisfied with the lack of "choice," and the model was mothballed. Since the overwhelming majority of patients receive their health insurance as a benefit of employment, the concept of paying for health care has become foreign. This, in large part, was the result of the enactment of Medicare as a health insurance for the elderly in 1965. In the mind of most patients, as well as most physicians, someone else is paying for this; therefore, the more tests the better. All headaches get an MRI, all bellyaches get a CT scan, and so on. Costs continued to spiral out of control, and as more and more diagnostics became available, they generated more and more billable events (1).

The accountable care organization model was developed as a bridge from our current fee-for-service method of financing care to a model that looks at outcomes, efficiency, and patient and provider satisfaction (2). While ACOs may not be the final endpoint of our evolving model, the tenets of the ACO directs us back to patient management and away from procedures and diagnostics. Another way of describing this change is that we must *care for* (and about) *patients*, and not focus on doing things *to* patients. The ACO can consist of multiple physician specialties or only primary care providers. However, the ACO must function as a solitary body, managing the comprehensive care of all patients, in order to be successful.

What Is Primary Care?

As mentioned above, primary care has undergone many changes over the years. It started as the family doctor who took care of everything and was always available. As specialties developed, the responsibilities of the primary care doctor decreased to essentially treating coughs and colds while referring all sick patients to the appropriate specialist. The HMO system made the primary care doctor into a sentry, blocking patients from seeing the specialist in order to control costs. Now we are attempting to reinvent the medical profession and create "value-based" compensation. The responsibility of the PCP, in this model, is to establish a preventive care program.

It is imperative to reconstruct the patient-provider interaction from a series of unrelated transactions to a long-term relationship. A person's health is a longitudinal, ongoing event, not a snapshot in time. There are periods of wellness and also episodes of illness. Some patients have chronic issues that alter the baseline and can increase the risk of adverse events. Some acute issues can be foreseen or mediated with early intervention. Sometimes there is no warning. The role of primary care is to participate with the patient through this journey. You need to assess every potential risk factor, be they genetic, environmental, congenital, or socioeconomic. You must develop a care plan for each and every patient, inclusive of all risks, historical events, and current treatments. This care plan is a living instrument, constantly updating in conjunction with the patient's experiences. It is your roadmap (or GPS) for their health care travel. How can this be done? Have you been trained to do this? Are the patients interested in this approach? Can you actually provide *health* care?

In the ACO, if you are the primary care provider, you are the face of the organization. You are responsible for interacting with all patients, at the least for the annual wellness visit (AWV). The AWV is encouraged by Medicare and paid for by them. It is during these visits that the majority of information is gathered by your team and incorporated into the patient's care plan. Updates to demographics, family history, medical history, medications, and allergies are gathered. Appropriate health screening is performed. The visit also serves as the glue that binds the provider-patient relationship. Appropriate education and teaching is performed at the AWV, as well as immunizations. Some patients with chronic illnesses may require more frequent visits, but an annual visit is the initial key to success. If the patient develops a relationship with you as the provider, then you can direct the diagnostic or specialty needs required by the patient. This is the reason that most approved ACOs are led by primary care physicians. In the past, PCPs have not had the same cachet as the specialists. Now it is clear that they are the logical leaders of ACOs. The PCPs should have the responsibility as the ACO leaders to analyze the clinical data and to minimize the variability of treatment. While care must be personalized, there are standards of best practice that must be adhered to. With many diseases, the variability of treatment can reach 50%, including unnecessary testing and substandard prescribing. The ACO leadership must provide education and oversight to minimize variation and improve outcomes and efficiency (3).

Who Is a Provider of Primary Care?

The historical model of medical care placed the physician as the provider of all services. An assistant may have administered treatment, but all decisions and recommendations were the responsibility of the physician. In the new model, it is clear that prevention, wellness, and minimizing severity of illness will be seminal in the control of costs. This requires all patients to receive care on a regular basis, in order to identify problems early, as well as to monitor and correct behaviors that are deleterious to health.

There are not enough physicians to perform all of these roles. A potential solution is the nurse practitioner or advanced nurse practitioner (APN), a registered nurse who has received postgraduate training in medical care and passed a licensing examination. An area of concern is the lack of standardization of training for APNs. While the curriculum is relatively standard, the only requirement for clinical experience is a letter from a physician stating that the student spent a specific number of hours at the office. While physicians must spend years of clinical exposure to become a primary care provider, APNs can potentially receive minimal training prior to certification. In most states, APNs can serve as PCPs and manage patients without direct supervision and can bill for their services. Therefore, it is important when selecting an APN that he or she has sufficient experience in a like setting. You should speak with the physicians the APN trained with. As critical is ensuring that your newly hired APNs are given adequate supervision. They should have sufficient time to orient with the physicians in your practice. There should always be a formal written evaluation of competence that is completed before the APN directs the care of patients unsupervised. While the addition of APNs as primary care providers is needed, we cannot afford to let the quality of care suffer. Therefore, part of the solution *must* be to standardize training and break down the walls between nursing and medicine.

Another potential solution to the problem of access to a PCP may be telemedicine. The technology to have real-time interaction between provider and patient via the internet exists and is improving daily. In areas such as behavioral health, where all interaction is by discussion, telehealth solves all access issues. However, examination is still an integral part of the provider-patient interaction in a PCP setting, and here telehealth displays its limitations. Screening, education, and follow-up can be managed in this manner. In our current state of fee-for-service, the compensation for a telehealth visit is still not resolved. As we move to other payment models, telehealth will become a vital cog in the relationship between patient and provider.

There are many other providers of care who must be considered primary care providers. Psychologists and clinical social workers provide counseling and support for many patients. Dentists and podiatrists commonly see patients with undiagnosed medical conditions. Physical therapists and nutritionists also play a vital role. It is apparent that primary care must be a team approach; however, there must be a captain of every ship. The ACO model requires a PCP or APN to be that captain.

Where is Primary Care Delivered?

Family doctors saw patients in their office, at the patient's home, or even in the physician's home. Over time this changed. Patients are now expected to come to the physician's office for appointments. If sick, there was no problem staying home from work and visiting the doctor. But for a minor ailment, a follow-up, or preventive care, patients were reluctant to lose a day's pay to go to the doctor. In addition, the practice was generally open only during regular work hours—a disincentive to seeking preventive care.

Due to their extended hours of operation, urgent care facilities have exploded on the landscape, commonly providing primary care to many patients. However, the care is fragmented, directed toward a specific complaint, and never preventative. Many pharmacies have opened "clinic" locations staffed by APNs to treat common ailments, provide immunizations, and conduct basic follow-up care such as blood pressure checks and diabetic glucose testing. While these different locations of care aim to fill a void, there is no continuity of care, care plans, education, prevention, or data collection. These alternate locations of care may fulfill minimal requirements of providing primary care, yet summaries of the visits need to find their way into the patient's medical record. As telehealth becomes more prevalent and ambulatory diagnostics are available for evaluation, the patient-centered medical home will be a logical location to integrate all this information. The patient-centered medical home is also an excellent location for education, which can be performed via telehealth.

As primary care moves toward providing more prevention service and early intervention, the majority of time spent in the past with the patient reviewing history, reconciling medications, and carrying out patient education and care planning will get short shrift. Much, if not all, of this process can be performed remotely in order to optimize face time between provider and patient. In addition, if payment is based upon outcomes, then frequent follow-up without evidence of progression of disease or noncompliance with treatment will become a joint obligation of patient and doctor.

ACOs must take ownership of the patient's health 24 hours a day, 365 days a year. Therefore, the care does not end when the patient leaves the office. The model must include regular interaction via text, email, phone, or video to ensure access to care at all times. Appropriate staff must be assigned to this process. Technology is a tool that can ease the burden of this responsibility, but technology is never a replacement for the human interaction.

What Services Are Needed for Success?

In order for primary care providers (and all providers of care) to optimize results, all pertinent information must be available for review. Our current state of personal health information is suggestive of the Tower of Babel. We have systems that do not talk to one another. Duplicate paper and electronic charts, false diagnoses, and multitudes of claims data has led to utter chaos. Various organizations use different data points to identify patients: social security numbers, medical record numbers, birthdates, names, and addresses. All information is manually entered, allowing for human error. Even within a single location of care, a patient may have multiple records if they provide slightly different information to registrars and health care staff. Examples include middle names, new addresses, marital status, and so on. In addition, if a patient requests their records to bring to a different provider, they routinely receive reams of paper with limited value. Aggravating the process is the request to pay for copying the chart.

All bills for service require a diagnosis code that accompanies a procedure code. For example, your patient undergoes a cardiac stress test in order to determine if symptoms are a result of coronary artery disease. You would put down the diagnosis code of "coronary artery disease." If the test is negative for any sign of coronary artery disease, the diagnosis remains the same. It is the same because payment depends upon a diagnosis rationalizing the procedure. Therefore, the patient has a bill documenting coronary artery disease that is received by the insurance company and placed in the patient's record. There is no mention of the test results in this database, only the test and the diagnosis. If the patient then applies for life insurance, he is told that he has coronary artery disease and is not eligible. This problem affects not only insurance applications but also risk stratification for premiums, care coordination, and resourcing of services.

There are programs being developed on a national level to create a digital solution for individual medical records. While this is a positive step, it will require all providers of care to participate, which may be costly and also time-consuming. Besides the benefit of having comprehensive information with which to plan care and decisions, a complete record can eliminate duplication of services and diagnostics, allow for accurate evaluation of gaps in care, monitor compliance and provider quality, and thereby lower cost of care.

The Role of the Team

It is obvious that primary care is not provided by an individual but by a team. Besides the primary care provider and appropriate support staff, the team must include a care coordinator (preferably a registered nurse as it is a clinical responsibility) and support from behavioral health, pharmacy, and educators. Currently, much of the effort within a primary care office is spent answering phones; making appointments; getting preauthorizations; calling insurers regarding covered services, denials, and payments; and coding, billing, and collection. None of these activities improves patient outcomes.

You can outsource most of these activities or eliminate many of them with alternative payment models. If the focus is on optimizing outcomes for all patients associated with a location of service, the primary care provider's office should look and function much differently. The organization responsible for the comprehensive care of patients would have a patient contact center, providing telephonic and digital support for all patients. All appointments would be scheduled there, including diagnostics, outpatient services, referrals, and planned hospitalizations. All transfers would be managed, including hospital-to-hospital, hospital-to-subacute, and subacute-to-home. Triage would be available at all times, allowing for direction to the appropriate place of service within the organization. All nonclinical services would be removed from the responsibility of the primary care office. A morning huddle would start the office day, with a review of all patients who are scheduled, potential gaps in care, and high-risk stratification. The need for other services, such as home care, education, dietary assistance, behavior modification, or family/caregiver conference, would be identified. Each member of the team would have a specific responsibility toward optimizing not only the visit but the continued interaction with the patient. We must eliminate the impression that the provider's responsibility ends when the patient walks out the door but instead continues ad infinitum.

Medication Management Is Often Overlooked

The importance of medication management in a primary care setting cannot be overemphasized. Many acute medical events are the direct result of medication interaction, adverse effects of medications, inadvertent or intentional noncompliance, and errors in prescribing or processing. Part of the value of a comprehensive electronic medical record is a real-time update of all medications filled, at any pharmacy and prescribed by any provider. You should address potential interactions. All possible adverse events must be documented. There are a multitude of medication reminder applications available for smartphones, and these should be reviewed by the primary care staff and by the pharmacy staff. All prescriptions must be documented, either by electronic submission or by printing a copy. In addition, we must eliminate pharmacy benefit managers from requesting automatic refills. This policy creates confusion when medications just show up in the mail without discussion between provider team and patient. We must focus on maintaining the provider-patient relationship at all costs, without external disruption by competing agencies. If we measure success by positive outcomes, patient satisfaction, *and* provider satisfaction, then the current model is a failure.

How Do We Pay for All This?

Inherent in the need for change is the fact that our health care financing model does not align with the goals outlined. We compensate providers for the things they do *to* patients not *for* patients. We compensate for *more* testing not *better* outcomes. We compensate for *more* patients hospitalized not preventing hospitalizations. We compensate *more* for a patient treated in an emergency department as opposed to an office location, no matter the diagnosis. Finally, we provide insurance to patients as part of employment or part of retirement benefits. Yet we allow the insurer to independently choose what medications will be covered. We allow Big Pharma to set any price they choose. Apparently, health care is a right that people demand of the government, yet insurance companies and pharmaceutical firms, inherent in the equation, are free from oversight. In addition, many companies prey on patients by offering medical equipment and supplies they may not require, simply by telling them "insurance will pay for it." In fact, insurance pays for little to nothing. They take the premium dollars that should be available to pay for patient care and freely distribute it to companies for services that the patient may not need.

Identifying Waste and How to Reduce It

It has been estimated that up to 25% of health care–directed dollars are wasted, meaning they do not contribute to patient care or outcomes. Consider duplicate or unnecessary services, testing, medications, treatments, and supplies. Even without changing the current system of providing care and compensating providers, we could cut the health care budget by up to 25%. All this waste has not even bought us improved outcomes or patient and provider satisfaction. Therefore, we must develop a new system as previously described. And we should start with where the majority of the spending is allocated, which is on inpatient hospitalizations. Many hospitalizations are the result of a lack of preventive care, noncompliance with treatment, and lack of education regarding healthy living choices. You should start there and then you will decrease the highest individual expenses.

A simple example of waste and misdirected care could be a case of chronic obstructive pulmonary disease (COPD). Following hospitalization for an exacerbation of COPD, patients are routinely given inhaled medication to continue treatment and prevent further episodes. Most of these medications are not approved by insurers or have very high co-pays. Your patients are being required to pay hundreds of dollars a month for the medication. It has been documented that the major cause of exacerbation in COPD is noncompliance with medication. Often it is because the medication is not affordable. It would be cheaper to pay for the medication rather than pay for repeat hospitalizations. Lack of alignment is the explanation for why this does not occur. A comprehensive primary care strategy combining prevention, education, compliance, and early intervention should decrease avoidable hospitalizations and assuredly decrease cost.

It is the responsibility of the ACO to oversee costs. This can be performed within a fee-for-service model, or preferably an alternative payment model. In a fee-for-service environment, insured patients, based on their diagnoses, have an estimated annual spend. If the ACO is able to decrease the actual spend, under the Medicare Shared Savings Program the ACO would receive a portion of the savings. Other alternative payment models take many forms, from global capitation to bundled payments. The ACO takes a certain amount of risk that their membership can bend the cost curve and decrease medical expenses. The ACO typically is not a replacement for the insurer, although some ACOs are trying to do that. If they sought that route, it might affect their ability to focus entirely on patient outcomes. The ability to improve quality performance and decrease expenses must be the criteria to sustain the work of the ACO. As in the Medicare ACO model, one must consider changes to provider compensation that will appropriately incentivize shared goals.

How Do We Negotiate Change with Insurers?

Our current model of health care financing depends upon the overwhelming majority of dollars being distributed by third parties. These can be insurance companies, third party administrators, corporations, or the government (local, state, and federal). When a service is performed, a bill is generated, and payment is made. Utilization review and preauthorization is a limiting factor that purportedly monitors and drives quality and minimizes waste. Each and every insured patient has a projected annual total spend based upon actuarial models and basic risk stratification. Premiums are adjusted based upon this expected spend. Premiums are adjusted up annually if a shortfall occurs. Government budget dollars to pay for care are based on similar calculations. The entire negotiating process with insurers has been based upon modification of payments made for specific services. There now is interest by insurers to negotiate population-based shared savings. This does not alter the fee-for-service payment but provides a bonus based upon unused dollars. While creating some physician attention to eliminate wasteful spending, this program is limited in its ability to change behavior and drive improved outcomes.

An affiliated model adds bundled payments for specific disease entities. An example is the joint replacement bundle. The cost of comprehensive care of the patient undergoing knee or hip replacement extending from the preoperative evaluation to 90 days post-discharge has been calculated. This includes professional fees, hospital fees, subacute care/rehabilitation, medications and supplies, and prosthesis cost. Organizations can agree to this single payment and distribute cost responsibility as it sees fit. The organization assumes the risk of unexpected care due to complications or noncompliance but keeps unused dollars if they are efficient and save. This model encourages efficiency and may change behavior, but liability is limited due to the limited time of responsibility. This model can be added to a shared savings model, or as a stand-alone. Theoretically, all isolated medical events, separate from surgical procedures, could be placed in a bundle. The concern is that prevention is not rewarded, because the bundle is only used if a patient suffers the medical malady.

Another model to consider is a global capitation model. This model provides the organization with the entire dollar amount for every patient's expected spend. This model drives the organization to prevent disease, or to perform early intervention. The payment model to the providers can be personalized. The risk involved is in building an appropriate system to minimize waste and provide close oversight of all patients. Having a stop-loss agreement, limiting potential loss, could mitigate this risk. Also to be considered are joint ventures with insurers to share risk as well as benefit.

No mention has been made of individual provider negotiations with insurers. This is because the model depends upon an integrated system that provides comprehensive care, either alone or with contracted suppliers, to manage populations optimally and achieve the best outcomes. In no way does it limit the ability to provide precision medicine to the appropriate patient or create bundles of care for specific diseases, nor does it deter primary prevention.

One must understand that health insurers are not in the health care business. They are in the insurance business. Therefore, it is up to the health care organization to drive quality metrics, indications for care, and best practices. Focus must always be on patients and their best interests.

How Does the Patient-Provider Relationship Change?

Our current system encourages transactions between patient and provider. You come in to the store for milk, and if the store proves convenient and friendly, you go back when you need milk again. No one checks on how the milk tastes, whether you are satisfied, or whether you need anything else. This is a mirror of current medical care in our country. We need to build relationships between the patient and the provider team. Relationships depend upon caring and trust. Our responsibility to the patient is ongoing and comprehensive. If they can't afford food, it's our problem also. If they forget their medication, we also suffer. If they refuse a treatment, we must be certain they understand all the risks and potential benefits. If that is the priority of all members of the treatment team, we will have been successful.

Part of this relationship is also the patient's responsibility. The trust must be bidirectional. If a patient is noncompliant, it may not be intentional. They must allow us into their lives so we can understand their difficulties, their needs, and their obstacles. If a child gets recurrent exacerbations of asthma despite compliance with medication, perhaps it is because his mother smokes in the house. All factors must be considered in order to be successful in this model. If a patient continues to make poor choices that adversely affect his health, perhaps there is a behavior issue that you need to deal with. Just as a cardiologist cannot be blind to all parts of the body besides the heart, a primary care provider cannot be blind to correctable external factors adversely affecting our patient's health, sometimes referred to as the social determinants of health. By interacting over many months and years, your relationship will continue to grow and prevention becomes the expected approach. Healthy choices become the norm. With each successive generation, our behaviors become ingrained in the expectations of the patient-provider relationship.

For ACO success, the provider-patient relationship must be reestablished and flourish. The best marketing is a happy patient. Without a successful relationship, all interaction is merely transactional, and care will suffer.

Conclusions to Drive Success

While primary care can exist without the ACO, your ACO cannot exist without the leadership of your primary care providers. An ACO's success must be measured by improved patient outcomes, increased efficiency, decreased treatment variation, improved patient and provider satisfaction, and reduced wasteful spending. The ACO membership must function as a single entity, assuming the responsibility for the health of the population it serves. While specialty services and hospital care are needed adjuncts to the total care of the patient, it is the primary care team that carries the burden of achieving overall success for the organization and health of the patient population.

REFERENCES

1. Rosenbaum L. Divided we fall. *New Engl J Med.* 2019;380(7):684–688.

2. Burgon TB, Cox-Chapman J, Czarnecki C, et al. Engaging primary care providers to reduce unwanted clinical variation and support ACO cost and quality goals: a unique provider-payer collaboration. *Popul Health Manag.* 2019;22(4): 321–329. http://doi.org/10.1089/pop.2018.0111.

3. Menacker M. Leadership's role in accountable care success: management in healthcare. *Am J Accountable Care.* 2018:6(3);166–173.

FOURTEEN

Practice Transformation

Engaging and Integrating Physician Practices

THOMAS KLOOS

Physician practice groups are typically certified as an integrated health care system by the Centers for Medicare and Medicaid Services (CMS) when you are approved as an accountable care organization (ACO). Many, in fact, are not integrated. Dr. Thomas Kloos provides a clear path for achieving real practice integration and physician engagement in order to become successful. He also warns of the competing government programs that may diminish an ACO's chance of survival.

Introduction

When I was asked to write a chapter for this book, and particularly around physician engagement and practice transformation, it admittedly gave me pause. Did we really have a kind of secret sauce to share with readers on becoming successful as an ACO, or were we just lucky? I do believe that it required certain foundational elements; the roots of our success were planted very early on. Optimus Healthcare Partners (OHP) became an accountable care organization in 2011 and began as a Medicare Shared Savings Program (MSSP) participant in 2012.

The genesis of OHP was an alliance between two independent practice associations in New Jersey: Vista Healthcare System IPA and Central Jersey Physician Network. These organizations had been active since the mid-1990s with commercial payers in pay-for-performance programs prior to the institution of the Affordable Care Act. Each independent physician association (IPA) was looking to develop the path toward clinical integration and found the accountable care organization concept consistent with such an approach. We made participation and membership in our ACO contingent on being a member of one of our underlying IPAs. By the end of 2017, OHP consisted of 206 primary care physicians and 289 specialists. We had developed a value-added contract with the MSSP, which had approximately 25,000 beneficiaries. In addition to the MSSP, OHP established value-based commercial contracts with all of the major payers in New Jersey and encompassed approximately 106,000 commercial beneficiaries.

Savings Achieved

Since beginning with the MSSP program, OHP's quality has improved over time, and patient satisfaction scores have remained consistently high. OHP has achieved a Medicare shared savings in every performance year, totaling an overall shared savings distribution of more than $23 million. Care management fees from our commercial value-added contracts have eclipsed $23 million. Since 2012, between these two revenue sources, OHP distributed over $28 million to the participants and members of Optimus Healthcare Partners as additional value-based payments.

The Engagement and Integration Process Begins

This begs the question: how did we get there? The main building block of our journey was physician recruitment. We were fortunate to have panels of physicians in both IPAs that had already been active to a small degree with previously described pay-for-performance programs. Nonetheless we recognized that performance in the new world of value-based contracts required a different mind-set from the traditional IPA model. Our initial staff was small and included two registered nurses assigned the role of population managers. Through collaboration with Horizon Blue Cross Blue Shield (BCBS) of New Jersey, we sent these nurses to undergo training at Duke University. Then we educated practitioners within a formal program setting to the concepts of population management. As our responsibilities grew, and recognizing our limited resources, we made a number of decisions that were to ultimately impact our potential for success.

Importance of Physician Champions and Strong Leaders Can't Be Overemphasized

One recommendation for successful ACO implementation is to mandate each practice joining a physician-led ACO to identify a physician champion within the practice as well as a clinical coordinator to interface with our ACO population managers. Yesterday's medical assistant became today's practice clinical coordinator without any new training or increase in salary. This gave us a starting point for engagement and training. Despite the rudimentary stages of the concept, it was a way to leverage practice resources to supplement our small staff. Based upon trust that we had developed with our partners in the IPA, physicians readily agreed to participate in our accountable care organization.

Secondly, we performed a practice assessment to understand where each partner was in the continuum of moving from fee-for-service to value-based care. To quantify these competencies, we developed an assessment tool to gauge practice readiness upon joining the ACO.

It was also extremely important for us to develop a solid culture. Early in our journey we were fortunate to have a strong leader in Dr. Jim Barr, a primary care physician who was also the president of the Central Jersey Physician Network and active in the patient-centered medical home (PCMH) movement nationally. Jim brought an omnipresent and all-encompassing passion toward messaging the value of this new health care transformation model. He quickly developed the motto "Care Better," and we embedded it into every one of our early presentations to physicians. The motto was also included on our webinar slides and all ACO documents.

Having a physician champion who has obviously bought into the value-based program is a must. Finally, we identified those physician leaders who would become our champions, to carry on the "Care Better" theme. They were our greatest advertisers and promoters. These physicians were engaged early on, helping to comprise our board of managers and our performance improvement and finance committees. Our mantra expanded to "We Help Physicians Care Better for Their

Patients," "We Help Patients Care Better for Themselves," and "We Help Individuals Care Better for Each Other."

One cannot understate the value of strong management talent. Our physician leadership included the previous medical staff president and revered local pediatrician Dr. John Vigorita, president and CEO of Optimus Healthcare Partners. The enterprise was also fortunate to have an exceptional operations officer in Deb Rodgers, MSN, RN, JD. Regulatory compliance with the varied rules in the Medicare Shared Savings Program can itself be a full-time job. CMS's new final rules that support the downside risk tracks within their Pathways to Success have made these requirements all the more complex. For example, they include the skilled nursing facility three-day rule waiver, the beneficiary engagement waiver, and a new notification policy.

Messaging the Goals

There is a risk of accountable care organizations getting too deep into their messaging around the financial aspects of these programs as well as the minute details of various quality reporting requirements. It is exceptionally important to continue to message that the real goal of what we do is to improve patient care: to reach out to populations of our patients who were not receiving our care and in the end to do what we all became providers for in the first place. It is critical to have a closer interaction with our patients: in other words, to care better. Our team and our supporters actively vocalized that message to our participants. To be successful as an ACO you need to keep this drumbeat going constantly.

Commercial Contracts Help Complete the Transformation

To be a successful ACO you cannot rely solely on the MSSP to generate enough interest from the physicians to undergo the transformational changes necessary. Another crucial decision on our part was the outreach to our statewide managed-care companies that were beginning to engage in the development of value-based programs.

As part of those contracts, payers offered up-front care management or care coordination fees on a per-member-per-month basis. These fees supported some of the costs involved in the basic infrastructure and transformational changes that practices needed to embrace. In 2012, Optimus completed contracts with Horizon BCBS, the largest and most progressive payer in this realm at that time within New Jersey, and we were able to distribute care management fees to our primary care physicians on a quarterly basis in support of transformational change. We also had a requirement within that contract stipulating that over 90% of our primary care offices would become certified as PCMH practices. While this was a somewhat onerous task, it was a valuable early transformational process. We would highly recommend having practices either being certified in or being held to the standards of the patient-centered medical home model.

After the signing of the Horizon contract, we rapidly developed and completed upside value-based contracts with each of the major payers in the state. We also felt that it was important that our ACO model was not considered just a pilot program. By bringing on commercial contracts, 50% of a physician's patients participated in a value-based program where the office was receiving care management fees. Presently, over 80% of our primary care physicians' patient panels are in a value-based program. This was not a pilot program but a transformational journey toward value-based reimbursements.

Financial Modeling

To be successful, an ACO needs to address the inevitable issue of "what's in it for me?" With our contracts in hand, we were able to show each primary care provider (PCP) what the shared savings opportunity would be based on:

- Attribution of patients within their practice
- Prediction of conservative savings below their ACO benchmark
- Projection of care management fees the practice would obtain from each of our commercial payers

Per Primary Care Physician   AACO Financial Proforma   Practice Attribution

	Maximum PMPM	2013 Potential Annual Amount	2013 Actual Paid Amount	2014 Potential Annual Amount	2014 Actual Paid Amount	Potential Shared Savings (Paid in 2015 for year) 2.5%	5%	7.5%
CMS								
Performance Improvement PMPM	$0.00	$0		$0				
Shared Savings						$21,319	$34,644	$47,968
						2013 and 2014 prepayments subtracted		
Payer 2								
Performance Improvement PMPM	$2.00	$2,400		$2,400		No shared savings		
Payer 3								
Performance Improvement PMPM	$4.00	No Contract		$33,600				
Shared Savings						$15,876	$25,799	$35,721
Final Shared Savings						–$17,724	–$7,802	$2,121
Payer 4								
Fully Insured PIIP PMPM	$2.40	No Contract		$2,880				
Self-Insured PIIP PMPM	$0.00	No Contract						
Shared Savings FI & SI						$11,794	$19,165	$26,536
Final Shared Savings						$8,914	$16,285	$23,656
Payer 5								
Performance Improvement PMPM	$4.00	No Contract		$12,000				
Shared Savings						$6,143	$9,982	$13,821
Final Shared Savings						–$5,858	–$2,018	$1,821

Practice Attribution:

	ACO Cost PMPM	Practice # Patients
CMS	$940	300
Payer 2		100
Payer 3	$300	700
Payer 4 FI	$325	100
Payer 4 SI		300
Payer 5	$325	250
Others		750
Total		2,500

Final Shared Saving are calculated by netting out the PMPM prepayments

	Potential 2013	Actual 2013	Potential 2014	Actual 2014	Potential 2014 Shared Savings: only MSSP negative balances are realized
Total PMPM Payments =	$2,400		$50,880		
Total Shared Savings =					$50,928 $75,565

TOTAL 2013	$2,400	TOTAL 2014	$50,880	+ 5% savings	$50,928	FINAL TOTAL 2014 =	$101,808
				+ 7% savings	$75,565	FINAL TOTAL 2014 =	$126,445

Figure 14.1. Financial opportunities in a typical primary care practice for value-based payments. The model combines practice attribution, care management fees, and various percentages in reduction to costs to illustrate the likely positive financial benefits.

This financial modeling, illustrated in figure 14.1, helped the PCPs to visualize the economic opportunities that these programs would bring to their practices. This was done at a time when payers no longer offered fee-for-service payment increases to our IPA participants via the messenger model. Recognizing that a payment shift was occurring in our markets, the other message we conveyed to our practices was that this was a way to work smarter and not harder.

Role of Education

Developing an active and ongoing educational program in population health is essential to ACO success. We believed this allowed us to be successful in the MSSP both early on and ongoing. In the beginning of our journey we set aside 45 minutes each Tuesday from 12:15 p.m. to 1:00 p.m. for an educational webinar. The topics were wide-ranging, including basics around the tenets of PCMH, population health, end-of-life care, appropriate diagnostic coding, annual wellness visits, and a litany of other themes. To date, we have currently completed and recorded over 200 webinars, and attendance has ranged between 150 and 170 online and live participants. We link participation in these webinars to our performance improvement incentive program. Additionally, we required each of our physician champions to participate in quarterly "provider-specific" webinars for information specific to our physician participants.

Developing strong relationships and an *esprit de corps* among clinical coordinators also is essential. At least twice a year, we sponsored meetings specifically for these crucial staff members. It was an opportunity to meet with one another in a social event where we could identify and applaud best practices while sharing this information across our practice groups.

How Did We Get Our Physician Practices to Engage in These Activities?

Practice transformation cannot occur without significant data transparency. A cornerstone of success is developing a robust data analytics team that produced key performance indicators for our primary care physicians. In our ACO, these reports were made available to every physician. In this manner we looked to capitalize on the intrinsic competitive nature of physicians: they do not wish to be last in their class.

For reports where protected health information was an issue, we posted information to a secure website. We used practice-specific folders containing reports on high-risk, high-cost patients; emergency room frequent flyers; and annual wellness visit rates. The folders also included integration reports that identified the activities occurring within and outside of our ACO. Medical directors within the ACO would also utilize these reports to develop focused action plans to present to each practice during at least one annual visit. This allowed for a frank discussion around opportunities for improvement as well as recognition of where the practices were doing great work. We also asked the physicians how we could share their best practices across the organization.

It is also worth mentioning the practical utility of early success in value-based programs—it delivers significant payments to offices undergoing transformation. In regard to distributing those payouts, the simple solution would have been to pay out equal amounts to each physician based on their beneficiary attribution. Instead, we took on the more challenging task of developing a performance-based architecture. It provided a financial payout of shared savings using following formula:

- 25% based on attribution
- 25% based on scoring within our quality measure set and citizenship metrics
- 25% based on the ability to bring their total per-member-per-month (PMPM) cost of care under the target that allowed us to get to shared savings
- 25% based on improvement in total medical cost trends throughout the performance year

The better a physician did within a particular category meant a larger component payment within that category. Shared savings distribution admittedly has been a double-edged sword because it has also become an expectation: an expectation that the same level of payments will occur in subsequent years. We found that when practices did not get the same level of payout, they voiced significant concerns. They forgot the fact that in any given year the vast majority of ACOs in this country did not receive any shared savings distributions.

Our Performance Improvement Incentive Program

While it can be debated that financial incentives to promote certain activities do not really work in the long run, at Optimus Healthcare Partners we found it to be an effective mechanism to stimulate process improvements and support our population health initiatives. We would recommend it to ACOs starting this journey. We have the ability to aggregate care management fees at the practice level. They vary based on the particular payer contract. We began early on to structure a quarterly performance improvement incentive program (PIIP). The program motivates the types of behaviors we felt would make us successful collectively as an ACO. We built the program around five pillars:

1. Care management and coordination
2. Population health management
3. Citizenship
4. Quality improvement activities
5. Engagement

We also formerly had an information technology category to stimulate uptake and usage of our population management software. The metrics within each of these categories would change on a quarterly basis in response to new directions we wanted to take. Based on a 100-point scoring system, practices would receive their entire care management payment for the quarter if they were to achieve at least 80 points. They would receive 75% of their commercial PMPM available if they achieved greater than 65 points, and they would receive 50% of their commercial PMPM if they achieved at least 50 points. No payment would be made if they did not submit an application or achieve at least 50 points.

The PIIP program is a dynamic tool that has evolved based on the requirements of our payer partners and the need to prepare our practices for greater financial risk. In the early renditions of the PIIP, practices could earn points for optional activities such as requirements to support the Merit-based Incentive Payment System (MIPS). The PIIP also focused on process improvements in quality. Today the PIIP has mandatory elements, such as an electronic medical record requirement. In our quality pillar, requirements have also shifted from a process (e.g., the demonstration of care plan development for a transitional care management visit) to an outcome, (billing for the visit where the ACO is able to validate activity via CMS claims data).

While we have seen some of our practices embrace the performance improvement program, others have not fully embraced the changes needed to work effectively in a value-based environment. We recognize that this is probably a mixed opportunity dependent upon the practices. We need to continuously upgrade the PIIP program and its metrics to support reengagement of those practices to the left of the bell curve. We conduct medical director outreach of these practices to offer peer-to-peer support. For our highest-performing practices that are already doing the right things for their patients, we have structured the PIIP program to be less burdensome administratively. Finally, practices that consistently do not submit their PIIP applications are requested to leave the ACO.

What Is the Main Factor that Made Us Successful?

What do we believe was the most significant end result that allowed Optimus to be successful in the MSSP five years in a row? When we review our quarterly expenditure and utilization reports, the one consistent standout area has been the PCP visits per 1,000 or how often our primary care practices are touching our Medicare beneficiaries. Throughout the years of success, Optimus practices had anywhere from 33% to 42% more primary care visits with MSSP beneficiaries than the national MSSP ACO average. If you see these patients more often at the PCP level, you better coordinate their care, close care gaps, and do all the right things to "Care Better."

Certainly culture development, education, financial incentives, and data transparency all contributed to this outcome as well.

Pathways to Successful Survival

Having had early success within the ACO model on predominately upside-only contracts, what does the future hold? I strongly believe that the ACO model is a foundational step in beginning the journey from volume to value and taking on downside risk. ACOs, as they move along this continuum, will develop a portfolio of initial upside-only contracts. Then, in subsequent commercial contract cycles, they will find that gradually more and more of the care management fees will be tied to performance-based quality and cost outcomes. As this occurs, and as the ACO continues to perform well in these settings, there is the natural progression to take on downside risk. Future opportunities, in both governmental and commercial programs, will be determined by what conflicting and competitive programs are developed by this and future administrations. The biggest risk to the ACO shared savings model is the development of overlapping models from the Center for Medicare and Medicaid Innovation. These include the bundled payment for care improvement advanced program, the oncology care model, and new mandatory bundles for cardiac services, among others. Since payers will not pay twice for shared savings, engaging specialists in these programs will help an ACO as long as there are still savings opportunities for the PCP in these models. Similarly, the Comprehensive Primary Care Plus (CPC+) initiatives as well as direct primary care programs in the future will further erode shared savings opportunities.

Can a physician-led ACO flourish among these models? In the short run, over the next five years, yes, while most hospital systems remain firmly entrenched in the fee-for-service, volume-based world. In the future, the winners in this space will be those partnering with health systems that understand the need to move to value-based care, who are willing and have the capital to underwrite the lion's share of downside risk repayment corridors, and who have the geographic footprints to allow for opportunities around narrow network Medicare Advantage programs and direct-to-employer contracting. We have been fortunate to have Atlantic Health System as a participant in Optimus Healthcare Partners since its inception to lend these levels of support and contribute their expertise, and whose current leadership under CEO Brian Gragnolati is leaning into the winds of value-based care. I do not see a wholesale movement to Medicare Advantage, but it will be a larger part of our contractual portfolio in the ACO as opportunities and enrollment continue to grow and competing programs continue to erode the MSSP.

I want to thank our entire initial Optimus team that helped us along this journey. This was the team that helped us build the plane with which we took to uncharted skies. This includes our initial tireless population management team of Deborah Eddy, RN; Annie Ryan, RN; and David Kloos. Our outreach assistant Laurie Hakim, RN, and our credentialing and network manager Bonnie Peacock. Since those early beginnings, our staff has grown significantly, and we now manage an additional health system–owned ACO. Despite such growth we remain steadfastly true to the tenets of "Care Better" and continue to place the provider and patient above all else.

FIFTEEN

Population Health Management Consulting

JOSEPH F. DAMORE

Joe Damore, as vice president for strategy, innovation, and population health at Premier Inc., describes his experiences as a consultant to many accountable care organizations. He emphasizes the importance of all providers—physicians and hospitals—moving in the same direction at the same time to be successful when implementing value-based care and payment changes. The discussion is rich in details on how to proceed and what to avoid along the way.

Introduction

Population health management consulting has grown rapidly since the passage of the Affordable Care Act in 2011. Many hospitals, physician groups, and health systems have been striving to learn how to implement effective core capabilities to successfully manage populations using value-based care tools and new value-based payment models. The assistance of seasoned consultants in this area can help you both speed implementation and avoid many pitfalls. The key is to use consultants who have extensive experience in implementing the core capabilities for successful population health management arrangements. And, in addition to implementing the core capabilities, successful consultants should also help you build a plan and improve performance.

Core Capabilities

There are eight key capabilities that are critical to implementing a successful population health management model, all which consultants can help implement:

1. Creating a strategic, operational, and financial plan to transform from a fee-for-service environment to value-based care and payment models
2. Developing an integrated system of care whose design involves and engages people, including patients
3. Operationalizing a robust team-based advanced primary care model and network
4. Managing high-risk and chronically ill populations with an effective care management program that is integrated with primary care practices
5. Building a high-value network that includes a post-acute care management system and integrated care with specialists who use evidence-based pathways, including clinical appropriateness criteria
6. Using a population health information management system that includes claims analytics, predictive modeling, care coordination capabilities, and a business intelligence tool
7. Employing a leadership and management team that includes the necessary clinical and administrative skills to successfully manage a population
8. Establishing new value-based payment arrangements that align payment with value rather than volume

Many organizations have struggled to make this transformation to value-based care and payment due to numerous factors, including the challenge of converting from a volume-based and acute care–based culture to a value-based culture focused on the full continuum of care. Others have struggled due to the lack of adequate resources to build these critical core capabilities. Many organizations have struggled with financial success as they strive to manage to live in both volume-based and value-based payment worlds simultaneously.

Successful organizations must transform both their care model and payment models in a synchronized manner to be successful (figure 15.1).

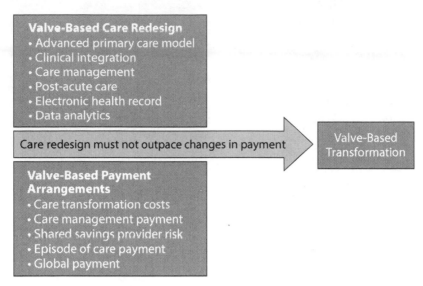

Figure 15.1. Integrating value-based care redesign and new value-based payment arrangements. Courtesy of Premier Inc.

A very progressive regional health delivery organization, which is a member of a large Midwest health system, transitioned to a value-based care model by building a team-based advanced primary care model. They also implemented an effective care management program and even began to build a high-value network that involved connecting with community agencies and organizations to help integrate the social determinants of health into their integrated system of care. However, the system was not able to change their payer contracts from volume-based agreements due to the fact that the system's corporate office negotiated all their payer contracts on a system-wide basis. It was a near financial disaster for this region until they were able to convince their corporate office to change their payment arrangements to value-based arrangements, even though nearly all the other regional systems continued with traditional fee-for-service contracts.

Another East Coast health system rapidly transitioned their payer contracts to value-based arrangements. They did not, however, effectively implement the care management and team-based advanced primary care model. The net result was also a near financial disaster.

Both situations demonstrate the importance of implementing value-based care capabilities and new value-based payment arrangements in sync.

Building a Road Map

Another major challenge for most organizations is how to determine the appropriate speed of the transition to value-based care and payment within both an organization and its market. A number of factors are used to help forecast the speed of change in a market. Figure 15.2 provides a brief overview of thirteen key factors, such as the organization of medical practice and payer readiness, that will help determine the speed of the transition to implement value-based care and payment models.

Building a plan and road map is the first step in this complex journey to population health management. First, complete an environmental assessment to determine the speed that the market will transform to

1	The organization of medical practices (small groups vs. large groups)		
2	The homogeneity/heterogeneity of the hospital and physician EMRs and their connectivity	8	The utilization patterns for health care services and the use of evidence-based practices
3	The medical community's culture based on concepts such as relationship and trust with each other and the hospital	9	The payer mix in the community, including reliance on commercial payers and fee-for-service Medicare
4	The current total per capita expenditure for Medicare and commercial beneficiaries	10	The organization's readiness for change and the financial stability of the health system
5	The supply, distribution, and model for primary care services	11	The core capabilities/infrastructure in place to manage the high-risk/high-cost and chronically ill populations
6	The readiness of payers to implement a value-based payment model	12	The level of transparency for key metrics such as quality and cost
7	The integration of the delivery system into organized contracting and delivery vehicles	13	The likelihood of existing or new, opportunistic competitors moving into value-based payment arrangements

Figure 15.2. Market factors determining the speed of transformation to value-based care and payments. Courtesy of Premier Inc.

value-based care and payment by considering many of the factors in figure 15.2.

An as example, two smaller health systems in a midsize southeastern community were assessing readiness of their markets for this payment transformation. Both independently decided to defer proceeding with the development of the core capabilities. They, unfortunately, did not realize that a large, independent primary care group in their market that referred to both hospitals was ready to move into value-based care and payment. The primary care group joined the Medicare Shared Savings Program (MSSP) Track 1, which included about 10,000 attributed Medicare beneficiaries. In their second year, they were able to reduce inpatient admissions by 20% to both hospitals. As a result, they enjoyed a multi-million-dollar shared savings check from the Centers for Medicare and Medicaid Services. Both hospitals, however, suffered volume and financial losses that led to significant volume declines and employee layoffs. It was an important lesson for these two organizations that used a less-experienced population health consulting firm for their market assessment.

A well thought out financial plan is also a critical part of the planning process. Many organizations overly invest in information technology and infrastructure too early in their journey. We urge you to use as many existing system resources as you can in the first years of this effort, such as finance staff, human resource staff, and so on. An expense plan that is tied to the contracting and revenue plan is critical for your success. The financial plan should not only include expense projections but also utilization changes as a result of implementing care management programs and revenue projections. Decreases in hospital admissions, emergency department visits, and skilled nursing facility admissions can lead to lower delivery system revenue, which must be offset by market share gains and expense reductions.

A three-year payer contracting plan usually starts with your own employee health plan and a Medicare accountable care organization (one-sided risk) in the first year. Many consultants divide the market into seven segments for purposes of developing a population health management strategy:

1. Employee health plan
2. Medicare ACO
3. Medicare Advantage
4. Medicaid-managed care
5. Uninsured
6. Commercial health plans
7. Direct-to-employer

A second part of the assessment is to determine the organization's current core capabilities that exist in a health system to implement a population health management model. A Premier capabilities framework assessment tool has been utilized in over 200 health systems across the country and measures 160 core operating capabilities necessary to successfully manage a population across all eight key capabilities noted earlier. Once these two assessments are completed, an implementation plan and a road map can be developed that includes a time frame, required resources, and priorities.

Once you have completed the plan and implementation road map, the role of the consultant changes from planning to assisting with implementation of these core capabilities. This includes the use of subject matter experts in each of the key areas, such as implementing advanced primary care models, care management, clinically integrated network development, population health information technology, and payer contracting specialists. The implementation time frame can be from 18 months to five years, depending on the market and organizational situation. The average implementation period is approximately three years.

Most organizations begin their journey by selecting one to three populations to manage as a learning laboratory. The conversion of the organization's employee health plan is usually a common starting point due to the fact that most organizations are self-funded and therefore at risk for their employee health care costs. A second common learning laboratory is Track 1 of the MSSP because it is one-sided risk only. A major benefit of this model is that MSSP participants will receive unblinded, timely, and comprehensive claims data for all Medicare Part A and Part B services for every beneficiary (except for behavioral health and substance abuse treatment). This will help your organization learn how to manage a population using claims data, which is critical to success. The expansion of the number of population health management arrangements and transitioning to two-sided risk models should be thought through carefully and planned. Success in one-sided risk models should be an organizational requirement before moving to two-sided risk contracts, which includes downside financial risk.

Performance Improvement

Finally, a key to success in this arena also includes the use of benchmarking data to measure cost, quality, network leakage, and utilization by provider. By benchmarking performance, consultants can help identify best practices that lead to better performance and assist in implementing best practices in areas such as emergency department visits per 1,000 beneficiaries and post-acute care costs per beneficiary per month. Implementation of performance improvement efforts is key to building sustained population health success.

Summary

The use of experienced consultants in population health management can provide a significant return on investment to an organization transitioning to value-based care and payment arrangements. Consultants experienced in operating integrated health systems, health plans, and physician-hospital organizations such as clinically integrated networks bring real world knowledge and expertise to your organization. Also, consultants who specialize in population health management can bring knowledge and examples of both keys to success and pitfalls to avoid.

Return on investment can result from assistance in focusing organizational efforts, reducing implementation time frames, and identifying the areas that will generate value to patients, providers, and organizations. The advice of experienced and knowledgeable consultants can save an organization significant time and resources in implementing a successful transformation to value-based care and payment.

SIXTEEN

The Comprehensive Primary Care Plus Initiative

SETH EDWARDS

Seth describes this new additional program that primary care physicians have joined to better manage their high-risk and chronic care patients. While this program pays additional funds, there are considerations and cautions when the Comprehensive Primary Care Plus Initiative is combined with the Quality Payment Program and the accountable care organization programs. This is a good example of how combining two Medicare programs can lead to unexpected issues.

Introduction

The Centers for Medicare and Medicaid Services (CMS) continue to develop value-based delivery system reform models to identify new approaches that are designed to improve the Triple Aim: improved quality, reduced costs, and improved patient experience. As a part of this initiative, CMS promulgated the Comprehensive Primary Care Plus (CPC+) Initiative, which began on January 1, 2017. CPC+ was created to build upon the foundational learnings gleaned from the Comprehensive Primary Care Initiative (CPCI), which was launched by the Center for Medicare and Medicaid Innovation (CMMI) in October 2012.

CMS characterizes the new model as "a national advanced primary care medical home model that aims to strengthen primary care through regionally-based multi-payer payment reform and care delivery transformation" (1). CPC+ is designed to test multiple payment mechanisms and care delivery approaches to determine if the model works to improve the health of the assigned population as well as reduce costs.

I should note for you that the precursor model, CPCI, experienced mixed results based on an analysis provided by Mathematica. Specifically, they found reports of improved delivery of primary care services related to care management, enhanced access, and coordination of transitions of care. In addition, certain aspects of Medicare spending were reduced. However, the report found the model did not reduce Medicare spending enough to cover the enhanced payments for the care management fee. The original model also did not improve patient or physician experience of care. Finally, compliance with Medicare claims-based quality measures did not improve (2). Based on these challenges, CMS and CMMI looked to develop a new model designed to address the challenges faced in the original.

CPC+ is also synergistic with the capabilities and approaches that will facilitate success in an accountable care organization. The approach to providing advanced primary care through a multidisciplinary team-based approach while incorporating the care redesign elements leveraged in this model poses a promising approach. However, before moving to join participation in CPC+ and a Medicare ACO model, there are specific considerations related to the success of the Medicare Shared Savings Program, the impact of payments from CPC+, and the impact on the Quality Payment Program in the Merit-based Incentive Payment System (MIPS).

Overview of the Comprehensive Primary Care Plus Model

With the CPC+ Initiative, CMS is testing programmatic elements that include payment augmentations as well as required care-delivery activities. CMS believes these changes will enable practices to invest in infrastructure to "deliver better care, resulting in a healthier patient population" (1).

Current Participation Numbers

As of publication, over 2,930 primary care practices are participating in CPC+. The program is not available nationally. Instead, CMS solicited interest through an application period from all types of payers from across the country. Based on the applications, CMS narrowed the program to 18 regions: Arkansas, Colorado, Hawaii, Greater Kansas City Region of Kansas and Missouri, Louisiana, Michigan, Montana, Nebraska, North Dakota, Greater Buffalo Region of New York, North

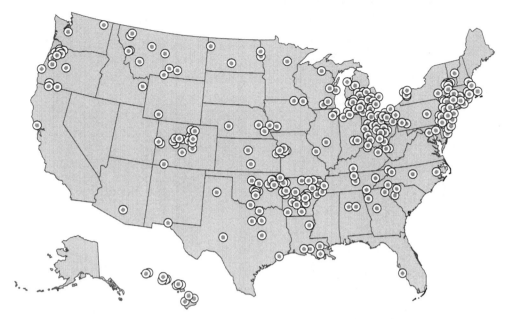

Figure 16.1. Comprehensive Primary Care Plus (CPC+) practices by region.
Courtesy of the Centers for Medicare and Medicaid Services.

Hudson-Capital Region of New York, New Jersey, Ohio and Northern Kentucky Region, Oklahoma, Oregon, Greater Philadelphia Region of Pennsylvania, Rhode Island, and Tennessee (1,3). Figure 16.1 outlines the geographic regions participating in the model.

Theory of Actions and Drivers

As you can see in figure 16.2, CMMI developed a visual of the CPC+ model as a driver diagram with five specific drivers:

Driver 1: Five comprehensive primary care functions
Driver 2: Use of enhanced, accountable payment
Driver 3: Continuous improvement driven by data
Driver 4: Optimal use of health information technology (IT)
Driver 5: Aligned payment reform

And each of these drivers has corresponding actions that are designed to alter caregiver behavior.

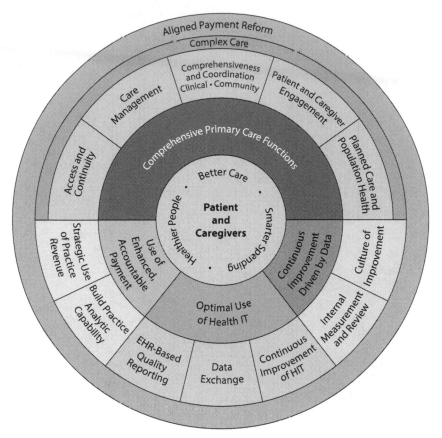

Figure 16.2. The theory of action for Comprehensive Primary Care Plus can be visually represented as a driver diagram. Courtesy of the Centers for Medicare and Medicaid Services Innovation Center.

Track 1 and 2 Segmentation

CPC+ is a five-year program with a two-tiered approach to engage with primary care practices. As you will see, the tiers are based on each practice's readiness for implementing comprehensive primary care. Track 1 is designed for practices that are earlier in their transformation process. Track 2 is designed for participants who have started to implement comprehensive primary care and are looking to increase the comprehensiveness of care through enhanced health IT and improve care of patients with complex needs. The requirements for practices to participate are outlined here.

Track 1 participation requirements
- o Certified electronic health record technology
- o Sufficient payer interest and coverage
- o Existing care delivery activities, which must include assigning patients to a provider panel, providing 24/7 access for patients, and supporting quality improvement activities

Track 2 participation requirements
- o Track 1 requirements
- o Existing care delivery must also include developing and recording care plans, follow-up with patients after emergency department visits, and implementing a process to link patients to community-based resources.
- o Letter of support from health IT vendor

Attribution Methodology

CMS developed an attribution method to assign patients to each practice in the new CPC+ model as well. This incorporates a prospective attribution methodology based on where a beneficiary receives the plurality of primary care service claims over the preceding two years. In order to receive attribution, the billing must have been tied to an internal medicine, general practice, geriatric, or family medicine specialty practice. The qualifying CPT codes used in the methodology are for

- office/outpatient visit evaluation and management services,
- complex chronic care coordination services,
- transitional care management services,
- home care,
- "Welcome to Medicare" and "Medicare Annual Wellness" visits, and
- chronic care management services.

This attribution methodology is very similar to the approach used in the Medicare ACO programs. The most significant difference is that the historical analysis looks back two years, while in the Medicare ACO programs, the analysis generally goes back only one year.

Payment Innovations

The second driver outlined is use of enhanced and accountable payment, which incorporates two principles: strategic use of practice revenue and building practice analytic capabilities. In order to achieve those goals, CMS has developed three payment models. Two of which are available to all participating practices and one that is only available to practices participating in Track 2. These payment models include a care management fee, performance-based incentive payments, and payment structure redesign through the Comprehensive Primary Care Payment.

Care Management Fee

Each practice participating in the program receives a quarterly, non-visit-based per beneficiary per month (PBPM) care management fee. The fee amount is determined by the number of attributed beneficiaries, the risk/acuity of the assigned population, and the track the practice is participating under. The rational for the acuity adjustment is that a practice serving more complex high-risk patients will need to provide greater amounts of care management. CMS estimates that participants in Track 1 will receive an average of $15 PBPM, and Track 2 participants will average $28 PBPM (including $100 PBPM to support patients with complex needs, such as dementia).

Performance-Based Incentive Payments

Paid at the beginning of each performance year, the performance-based incentive payment is then retrospectively reconciled and dependent on how the practice performs on quality, utilization, and patient experience measures. Performance-based incentive payments are included for both CPC+ tracks. Practices in Track 1 will receive $1.25 PBPM for quality and patient experience of care measures and $1.25 PBPM for utilization performance. Track 2 practices receive a higher amount of $2 PBPM for both portions of the payment.

Comprehensive Primary Care Payment

While practices will continue to be paid via the Medicare fee-for-service (FFS) model, participants in Track 2 will receive a hybrid payment between FFS and an upfront lump-sum payment. The lump-sum payment, known as the Comprehensive Primary Care Payment (CPCP), is distributed quarterly. It is based on historical FFS evaluation and management billing. The CPCP is designed to be approximately 10% greater than the historical annual PBPM billing for the practice, as it is expected to counterbalance the increased breadth and depth of services required by the model. CPC+ practices are able to select how rapidly they want to move to the CPCP model and are able to select a range between 10% CPCP/90% FFS to 65% CPCP/35% FFS.

Multi-payer Approach

In addition to the Medicare payer participation, CMS created this model as a multi-payer program and opened applications to all other payers, from Medicare Advantage plans and Medicaid state agencies to self-insured businesses. The rational for this approach is to create a critical mass of reimbursement tied to a value-based model and for practices participating in the program to transition to this payment and care delivery method.

Participating payers are required to offer

- enhanced non-fee-for-service support,
- a change in cash flow mechanism from fee-for-service to at least a partial alternative payment methodology,
- performance-based incentives,
- aligned quality and patient experience measures, and
- practice- and member-level cost and utilization data determined at regular intervals.

In addition, participants are required to complete a number of activities throughout each performance year, which gradually lead to comprehensive primary care and fall into five categories:

- Access and continuity
- Care management
- Patient and caregiver engagement
- Planned care and population health
- Comprehensiveness and coordination

There are a number of activities that roll up to each of these five areas. For the first year of the program, depending on the track and prior participation in the CPC model, practices were required to complete between 13 and 24 required activities. The expected number will increase over time.

Quality Reporting Requirements

CPC+ practices are required to report quality metrics on a quarterly basis. The performance period for each year aligns with the calendar year. As of publication, there are 14 electronic clinical quality measures associated with the program. CPC+ practices must successfully report 9 of the 14 measures annually, with reporting required at the practice site level. CPC+ practices must select from two of the three outcomes measures, two of the four complex care measures, and five of any of the remaining measures.

Interaction with the Quality Payment Program

As of publication, CMS has deemed that CPC+ qualifies as an advanced alternative payment model (Advanced APM) for the Quality Payment Program (QPP). This classification allows participants to opt-out of MIPS, assuming they meet certain threshold requirements related to revenue or patient count going through the model. Figure 16.3 outlines the threshold requirements, which are aligned with the year that payment will be impacted. Qualification as an Advanced APM participant guarantees a 5% bonus payment on the practice's Part B billing (4).

Under current rules, all CPC+ participants who are not in a Medicare ACO are able to qualify as an Advanced APM participant. In the

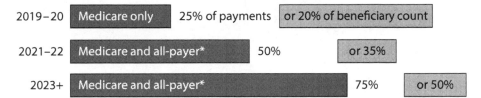

Figure 16.3. Threshold of payments and/or beneficiaries in an advanced alternative payment model to reach quality payment status. *All-payer option: Minimum of 25% of Medicare payments must be in the advanced alternative payment model (AAPM) in all years for quality payment (QP) and 20% for partial QP. Bonus only for QP and MIPS exempt. No bonus for partial QP and MIPS exempt, unless AAPM elects to opt in to MIPS.

original Quality Payment Program rule, CMS created a provision that can limit the applicability of the Advanced APM status to entities comprised of, or owned by entities comprised of, less than 50 eligible clinicians (4). This provision was designed to push larger organizations to accept greater amounts of risk. The 2017 QPP final rule removed the implementation of this rule for a year; however, CMS may implement it in the future.

Considerations and Implications for Dual Participation

As we discussed at the beginning of the chapter, while the Medicare ACO model and CPC+ are very synergistic, there are a number of considerations related to participating in both programs. The first set of considerations is related to the impact on the CPC+ program, the second is related to the QPP, and the third is the impact on the Medicare ACO programs.

CPC+ Considerations

While CPC+ practices are able to concurrently participate in the Medicare Shared Savings Program, there is an impact related to the payment adjustments included in the model. Specifically, dual participants are unable to receive the prospective performance-based incentive payment.

In place of these payments, practices are able to potentially share in the savings achieved by the ACO.

Quality Payment Program Considerations

Since CPC+ is considered an Advanced APM for the Quality Payment Program, and because of the change in the performance-based incentive payment for dual participants, the model no longer qualifies as an Advanced APM for practices also participating in a Medicare ACO. Instead, the QPP designation reverts to the Medicare ACO's track. Risk-bearing ACOs in Tracks 1+, 2, and 3 qualify as Advanced APMs. ACOs participating in Track 1 are considered MIPS APMs.

Medicare Shared Savings Program Considerations

In addition to the QPP consideration outlined above, there are other impacts on the Medicare ACO. Specifically, each of the additional payment enhancements included in the CPC+ model will count against the ACO's expenditure calculation, and it is often not included in the benchmark calculation. While these payments create incentives for practices to align with the goals of the ACO, it can create a dynamic that can make achieving shared savings challenging for the ACO.

Summary

As CMS continues to promulgate new rules and models, it is important for organizations to evaluate and strategically assess the opportunity to participate. Due to overlap and interaction, participating in multiple models can be challenging and the impact can be unclear—even if the models appear to be congruent. The CPC+ model is a great example of this overlap. The program provides upfront payment that practices can use to invest in developing capabilities that will facilitate success not only in CPC+, but also in an ACO model. With that said, these payments can have an impact on the ability for the ACO to successfully achieve shared savings. Caution and consideration when making selections is the byword.

REFERENCES

1. Comprehensive Primary Care Plus. Centers for Medicare and Medicaid Services website. https://innovation.cms.gov/initiatives/comprehensive-primary-care -plus. Accessed June 17, 2018.

2. Peikes D, Dale S, Ghosh A, et al. The Comprehensive Primary Care Initative: effects on spending, quality, patients and physicians. *Health Aff (Millwood)*. 2018;37(6):890–899. doi:10.1377/hlthaff.2017.1678.

3. Comprehensive Primary Care Plus: based on CMS Innovation Center model participants. Data.CMS.gov website. https://data.cms.gov/Special-Programs -Initiatives-Speed-Adoption-of-Bes/Comprehensive-Primary-Care-Plus/eevd-hiep. Accessed June 11, 2018. Updated October 3, 2019.

4. Centers for Medicare and Medicaid Services. Medicare program; Merit-based Incentive Payment System (MIPS) and alternative payment model (APM) incentive under the physician fee schedule, and criteria for physician-focused payment models. *Fed Regist*. 2016;81(214):77008–77831. To be codified at 42 CFR § 414, 495. https://www.federalregister.gov/d/2016-25240/p-4906. Accessed June 12, 2018.

SEVENTEEN

Keys to Success in Bundled Payments

MARK HILLER, BETH IRETON, MIRIAM MCKISIC,
AND MIKE SCHWEITZER

Bundled payment programs offer a more narrow focus on cross-continuum care delivery for episodes as compared to an accountable care organization's population-wide focus. Bundle programs can provide a potentially complimentary strategy, however, due to the typical subspecialty focus of bundles as compared to the typically more primary care focus of accountable care. Mark, Beth, Miriam, and Mike show how both can work together. Bundled payments concentrate on a specific disease or procedure. For example, renal failure, oncology, or bone procedures such as hip and knee replacements. How to manage this approach is well described by the authors. In addition, the new Bundled Payment for Care Improvement (BPCI) Advanced is considered.

Introduction

In our current health care environment, fee-for-service pressures are pushing commercial and government payers, health systems, and other providers to pursue new, alternative payment options for competitive advantage and economic survival (1). Bundled payment models represent both a unique and attractive alternative to fee-for-service, creating new opportunities to work to improve quality and manage costs. At the same time, opportunities are created for providers to earn new revenue in the form of shared savings.

You might be surprised to learn that bundled payments have a long, diverse history dating all the way back to the 1980s. Through numerous tests of change, research has shown that creating financial incentives for care across an episode of care is an effective strategy for improving patient outcomes. It enhances care coordination and aligns providers behind shared performance improvement goals (2). The Medicare bundled payment models have been an early leader promoting adoption of bundled payments. Now many commercial payers have also implemented these types of alternative payment models as a strategy to effectively incent change.

You can implement bundled payments as a vital strategic tool if you are just beginning the journey toward value-based care. On the other hand, global payments or accountable care organizations (ACOs) require an organization-wide mobilization and also the potential assumption of downside financial risk that many find daunting. Bundled payments can be tested within a few services lines (or even for a condition within a single service line) and expanded gradually to other service lines if successful. Bundled payments can also be aligned with evidence-based clinical guidelines for cost and quality improvements, making the effort very focused. Lastly, you can use bundled payment models to create incentives to bring in providers that are traditionally left out of ACO or primary care–based models. These other providers include specialists and post-acute care providers that can have a major impact on your total spending as well as patient outcomes.

Despite its appeal as a fairly broadly utilized and focused model by Medicare and some commercial payers, bundled payment models can't be entered into without risk. There are a myriad of model participation selections and care episodes that can be chosen. They each require a careful analysis of your data, existing infrastructure, and/or contract requirements to identify episodes that provide the most viable options to improve your organization's patient outcomes and financial success. Moreover, bundled payments also require you to have an ability to align with provider partners across the continuum. You have to identify engagement and incentive structures that will promote the right amount of change at the right pace and then refine them on an ongoing basis. You are also required to measure cross-continuum performance through analysis of claims, data, provider performance, financial, and outcomes data. Most importantly, care management needs to be integrated into an overall program of clinical transformation with full leadership backing.

Bundled payments do require very specific clinical, technical, and administrative capabilities across the care continuum. When executed properly, they create opportunities for providers to leverage greater financial incentives while improving care delivery practices. At the same time, patients, payers, and employers reduce expenses by avoiding unnecessary services and health care complications while realizing better outcomes. As these models continue to take hold, you must be skilled at assessing opportunities and managing risk. You will be evaluating readiness, identifying opportunities, and implementing cross-continuum changes to the delivery system. In the process, you will have created an infrastructure for ongoing management and measurement. These are just a few of the key pillars for success.

Growth and Benefits of Bundled Payments
Medicare Bundled Payment Models

Medicare has been experimenting with bundled payment models for many years. Since 2013, Medicare has been implementing bundled payment programs broadly with the expectation of improving care while reducing costs. In the last five years, Medicare has launched four bundled payment models:

- o Bundled Payment for Care Improvement (BPCI), started in October 2013
  Model 1: Retrospective acute-care hospital stay only
  Model 2: Retrospective acute and post-acute care episode
  Model 3: Retrospective post-acute care only
  Model 4: Prospective acute-care hospital stay only
- o Comprehensive Care for Joint Replacement (CJR), started in January 2016
- o Oncology care model (OCM), started in July 2016
- o BPCI Advanced, started October 2018

More than 1,600 organizations have participated in the legacy BPCI model, taking on risk for more than 14,000 clinical episodes (3). An additional 465 are participating in the Medicare CJR program (4), and 187 practices have joined the OCM (5). The latest model, BPCI Advanced, will further grow bundled payment participation on a national level, giving both existing and new entrants experience in the value-based payment environment. This growth is being driven by the significant savings that bundling has been able to generate.

BPCI evaluations indicate that bundling has been effective in improving quality and reducing overall costs. According to current program analysis, Medicare payments for joint replacements decreased an average of $1,273, or 4.5%, per case among BPCI participants Similarly, congestive heart failure spending dropped by an average of $970 per case, or 3.6% lower than the baseline (6). In addition, 47% of all participants in the CJR program achieved savings, earning $37.5 million in added Medicare shared savings payments (7).

Non-Medicare Bundled Payment Models

Outside the Medicare program, you can find hundreds of other bundled payment initiatives existing in the private sector (e.g., commercial). More than 20% of employers contract for bundled payments directly with providers (8) through their private health plans. These contracts include organizations such as Boeing, Walmart, Kroger, Lowe's, and PepsiCo (9). Commercial payers also have other bundled payment models in place, with dozens of bundling initiatives across the country, particularly among Blue Cross Blue Shield plans (9).

Benefits of Participating in Bundled Payment Models

By participating in a bundled payment model, you can expect a range of revenue, cost, quality, and patient care improvements.

Aligned incentives
The driving factor steering provider interest in bundled payments is the alignment it creates between hospitals, physicians, and other providers. Traditionally, hospitals paid under the Medicare Severity-Diagnosis Related Group (MS-DRG) system were highly motivated to reduce any unnecessary expense in order to optimize margin, while physicians paid under the fee-for-service model had little exposure to the cost of their

services. A similar phenomenon exists among post-acute and other providers, leaving very few caregivers accountable for total costs. Bundled payments inject the same level of price sensitivity into all clinical decision-making and promote shared accountability for costs, quality, and outcomes. Bundled payment models that are supplemented with gain-sharing or other bonus programs for eligible physician providers create greater incentives for active physician participation. It clearly raises awareness of episode costs throughout the continuum of care.

Improved clinical performance
Because you can have financial consequences attached to errors or deviations from evidence-based practices, many bundled payment participants begin their journey by standardizing care to guidelines and post-discharge procedures. They hard wire the standards into every clinical interaction. As best practice becomes the standard for care, clinical quality typically improves across the board. In particular, standardized care has been shown to improve clinical quality in a number of high-visibility areas. Finally, standardized care has been particularly effective at reducing complications, infections, and readmissions (10).

Improved financial performance
For many procedures, you will find wild variation in total costs. For instance, research shows that per episode, payments to highest-cost hospitals were higher than those to the lowest-cost facilities by up to $2,549 for colectomy and $7,759 for back surgery (11). Bundled payments incent providers to work together to compress that variation by allowing providers to receive a portion of the episode savings generated. These funds can go straight to the bottom line or be used as an investment in further improvement efforts.

Value-based payments extended to specialists and post-acute care
Many value-based or population health models, like ACOs and patient-centered medical homes, are heavily focused on optimizing disease prevention and overall health to avoid costly health care utilization. As such, the focus is heavily skewed toward primary care services. Bundled payments, however, target surgical services and recovery and/or exac-

erbations of medical conditions. In addition, they create participation incentives for specialists and other providers, adding to the total cost-savings potential. For instance, post-acute care and readmissions account for nearly 40% of Medicare spending for 30-day cardiac care episodes and 37% for spending on joint replacement episodes (3). Better management of post-acute utilization represents a major savings opportunity for bundled payment participants, and it can help you optimize performance across all value-based care contracts.

Alignment to other transformation initiatives
Bundled payments can be a strategy for success within a range of clinical and financial improvement initiatives. If you are still predominantly in the world of fee-for-service, optimizing performance in select surgical procedures or medical episodes can help. It can help you avoid financial penalties tied to complications or overall system readmission rates. If you are in an ACO, bundles can help you reduce overall spending among specialists and post-acute providers, generating further cost savings that return to the providers in the form of percentage-based shared savings payments. In addition, bundles can be an effective strategy to ensure alignment and successful performance under the Quality Payment Program (QPP) of the Medicare Access and CHIP Reauthorization Act (MACRA) of 2015. The QPP ties physician payments to quality indicators and provides additional upside payments to those that participate in two-sided risk-bearing bundles. By coordinating with ACO teams and efforts on post-acute care, bundles can be a synergistic strategy to employ with ACOs.

Competitive differentiation
Because bundled payments have the potential to improve patient outcomes in addition to generating significant savings, your participation in any of the models can be a competitive differentiator. Particularly in crowded, competitive metro markets, providers are increasingly being driven into alternative payment arrangements in order to provide better care (and prove it), manage margins with additive shared savings payments, and retain high-value physicians through financial alignment and by enabling their success within MACRA.

Providers that aren't preparing to take advantage of these opportunities risk losing market share to competitor organizations. In addition, be aware that inclusion in narrowed payer networks increasingly only occur with high-value health care organizations.

Overview of Bundled Payment Models
How Medicare Bundled Payments Work
Episode definition
Since bundled payments pay for all care treatment within a defined episode of care, most models begin by defining the diagnoses and services to include in the bundle. Your episodes are generally grouped into procedural or medical families that include almost all services provided to patients receiving similar procedures or with similar diagnoses.

Target price
Your target prices are derived from program- or contract-specific methodology for calculating spending per episode. Target price calculations usually include the organization's historical spending, can include or be based solely on regional spending, and typically include additional modifiers or adjustments depending on the model. Understanding the composition and methodology used to derive target prices is critical to evaluating your opportunity for success.

Payment
You are typically paid via traditional fee-for-service reimbursement (e.g., retrospective model). After a period of time to allow for claims runout, payers look back on your actual costs and quality outcomes. If your quality metrics are met and the total spend is less than the target price, the payer will send a certain percentage of the savings back to you as a participant (typically the risk-taking participant). If total spend is not less than the target price, you may have to pay back the difference to the payer. In the case of government-led models, the payer is the Centers for Medicare and Medicaid Services (CMS) (i.e., downside financial risk).

Risk corridors

Most of the CMS bundled payment models include stop-loss and stop-gain limits at both episode and aggregate levels, giving you financial protection from outlier cases or performance periods.

Quality requirements

The latest Medicare bundled payment models (i.e., CJR and BPCI Advanced) require achievement of certain quality metrics in order for you to be eligible for savings payments through reconciliation. This aspect, along with satisfying certified electronic health record technology requirements, allows for the models to be eligible as MACRA advanced alternative payment models (Advanced APMs).

Exclusions

Most Medicare bundled payment programs include Parts A and B services provided during the episode, including hospital care, physician care, readmissions, post-acute care, and durable medical equipment, less certain exclusions defined by the program. Current models such as BPCI, CJR, OCM and BPCI Advanced have episodes that exclude certain readmissions and Part B services that are unrelated to the index admission, including services such as transplantation, trauma services, acute surgical procedures, and cancer admissions. Figure 17.1 outlines the general structure of a typical bundled payment model.

Oncology Care Model

On February 12, 2015, the Center for Medicare and Medicaid Innovation announced the launch of a bundled payment model that focuses on cancer patients. The Oncology Care Model gives you episode-based payments to incentivize further-coordinated and efficient outpatient chemotherapy care for physician practices and some payers. Approximately 200 physician groups and 17 payers participate in the OCM (12).

With more than 1.6 million people diagnosed with cancer in the United States each year (of which, 50% are Medicare beneficiaries), cancer patients comprise a medially complex and high-cost population (13). The goals of the OCM line up closely with previous models before it:

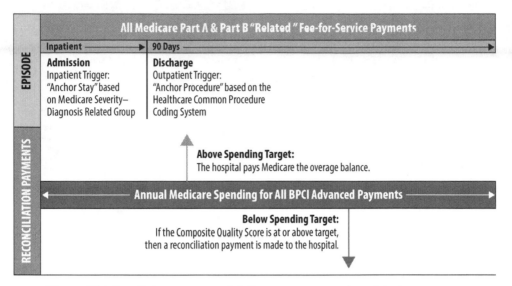

Figure 17.1. Bundled-payment model diagram representative of the latest model, BPCI Advanced; however, Bundled Payment for Care Improvement (BPCI), Comprehensive Care for Joint Replacement, and the Oncology Care Model follow this construct very closely as well. Composite Quality Score adjusts total reconciliation by up to 10% based on relative performance. Target price is a 3% discount based on historical target. Courtesy of Premier Inc.

to support better quality care, promote positive health outcomes, and safely lower costs for those patients undergoing chemotherapy.

This model is set to run for five years and began on July 1, 2016, for Medicare fee-for-service (FFS) beneficiaries. Similar to other CMS bundled payment models, the OCM is a retrospective model, which allows for FFS payments to occur during the episode, then savings or repayment is made based on performance compared to a target price.

One of the unique factors in the OCM is its six-month episode duration (BPCI had 30-, 60-, or 90-day episode options, and CJR and BPCI Advanced require 90-day episodes). These episodes include all cancer diagnoses treated with oral or IV chemotherapy. No downside risk is required initially. However, there is an option for you to elect for downside risk in performance year three in order to qualify as an Advanced APM under the MACRA ruling.

To further incentivize cross-collaboration, the OCM incorporates a unique (to Medicare) payment mechanism called a monthly enhanced oncology services (MEOS) payment valued at $160 per patient. This is in addition to a performance-based payment tied to quality measure adjustment. If your "actual" Medicare FFS spending plus the MEOS payment comes in below the spending target set by CMS, then a positive payment (which includes a positive or negative quality adjustment) is given back to you (e.g., physician practice). If a beneficiary is attributed to both the OCM and CJR or BPCI Advanced, the OCM performance-based payments will be adjusted for CJR or BPCI Advanced performance.

CMS outlines certain requirements for the OCM, as follows:

- Allow 24/7 patient access to an appropriate clinician who has real-time access to patient's medical records.
- Use an Office of the National Coordinator for Health Information Technology–certified electronic health record and attest to Stage 2 of meaningful use requirements.
- Provide core functions of patient navigation.
- Document a care plan for every OCM patient that contains the 13 components (table 17.1) in the Institute of Medicine Care Management Plan. These care plan elements can be in multiple places within the electronic health record so long as all are accessible to the care team.

Table 17.1. Thirteen components of the Institute of Medicine Care Management Plan

1. Patient information
2. Diagnosis
3. Prognosis
4. Treatment goals
5. Treatment plan
6. Expected response to treatment plan
7. Short- and long-term treatment benefits and/or harms
8. Quality of life and likely experience with treatment
9. Care coordination with other care teams
10. Estimated financial costs
11. Advance care plans
12. Psychosocial health needs plan
13. Survivorship plan

- Treat patients with therapies consistent with nationally recognized clinical guidelines (American Society of Clinical Oncology, National Comprehensive Cancer Network, others to be approved by CMS). Exceptions, such as clinical trial participation, must be noted in the electronic health record.
- Utilize data for continuous quality improvement. Quality measure areas come from several sources and fall into three categories (figure 17.2).

In conclusion, various key OCM success strategies include

- reduced variability in treatment plans;
- reduced excess utilization, as appropriate;
- closely monitoring inpatient admissions/readmissions, emergency department visits, imaging, and other ancillary services;
- evaluating post-acute care settings (e.g., skilled nursing, reduced drug expense);
- increased palliative care/hospice utilization, as appropriate;
- improved patient navigation/care coordination; and
- medical records documented comprehensively and appropriately.

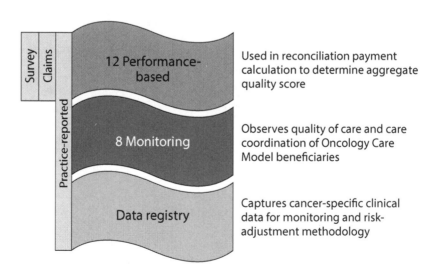

Figure 17.2. Quality measures for the Oncology Care Model (OCM). Courtesy of Premier Inc.

Comprehensive Care for Joint Replacement

The CJR program is a retrospective, two-sided risk model with hospitals bearing financial responsibility for eligible Medicare beneficiaries. Participation is mandatory in 34 select metropolitan statistical areas (MSAs) and voluntary in 33 MSAs for the inpatient prospective payment system and does not include hospitals entered into the second application period of models two or four of the original BPCI initiative for lower joint clinical episodes. The CJR program is expected to save Medicare over $200 million in just the last three years of the model duration (14).

The CJR episode consists of Medicare Part A and Part B fee-for-service payments beginning with hospital admission and ending at 90 days post-discharge specific to the following diagnosis-related groups:

- MS-DRG 469: Major joint replacement or reattachment of lower extremity with major complications or comorbidities
- MS-DRG 470: Major joint replacement or reattachment of lower extremity without major complications or comorbidities

In most cases, Bundled Payment for Care Improvement takes precedence over CJR episodes during the life of the BPCI program. For example, BPCI-related major joint replacement episodes that overlap with Comprehensive Care for Joint Replacement episodes will take precedence over the CJR episodes. In addition, if a BPCI major joint hospital participant resides in a mandatory CJR metropolitan statistical area and dropped out of the BPCI model, the hospital would be subject to the CJR model. Upon the conclusion of the BPCI program, lower joint clinical episodes that had been in BPCI will become part of CJR. CJR will have precedence over BPCI Advanced for the remaining life of CJR.

The type of services that are included within CJR episodes include

- physicians,
- inpatient hospitalization (including readmissions),
- inpatient psychiatric facility,

- long-term care hospital,
- inpatient rehabilitation facility,
- skilled nursing facility,
- home health agency,
- hospital outpatient services,
- independent outpatient therapy,
- clinical laboratory,
- durable medical equipment,
- Part B drugs, and
- hospice.

Similar to the previous bundled payment models discussed, you would continue to bill and receive reimbursement according to the current FFS structure, as they do today. At the completion of the performance year, actual claim spending is compared against the episode target price. You may receive a reconciliation payment if the quality thresholds have been met and actual spending is less than the target. Hospitals are responsible for paying Medicare for actual spending greater than target up to certain caps. The maximum required discount factor is 3% and this discount factor may be reduced depending on quality performance. Downside risk is phased in during performance years two through five with no downside risk in performance year one (PY1). Participating hospitals receive projected target pricing prior to each performance period for each MS-DRG.

Your target prices within CJR are based on three years of historical data and are updated every other year. Target prices began as a combination of hospital-specific and regional (by US census region) historical payments and transitioned to regional-only rates (figures 17.3 and table 17.2). This blended and prospective target price concept is different from the original BPCI model. Your reconciliations occur once per year compared to quarterly in BPCI. There was also phased-in risk for CJR participants. No downside risk occurs in performance year one, then downside risk is phased in for performance year two, and finally it ends in full downside risk in years three through five.

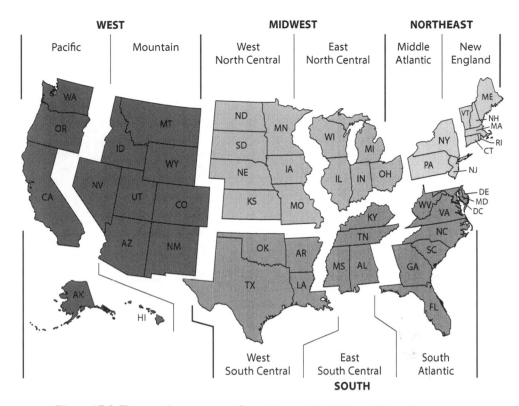

WEST

Pacific | Mountain

MIDWEST

West North Central | East North Central

NORTHEAST

Middle Atlantic | New England

SOUTH

West South Central | East South Central | South Atlantic

Figure 17.3. Target price census regions. Courtesy of the US Energy Information Administration.

The quality scoring within comprehensive care for joint replacement is also a new addition as quality scoring was not a part of the original BPCI model. Overall quality performance for CJR is measured on a 20-point scale according to percentile performance for the risk-standardized complication rate, the Hospital Consumer Assessment of Healthcare Providers and Systems (HCAHPS), whether hospitals choose to report the voluntary patient-reported outcomes measure(s). There are three terms that are used in the intermediate steps to determine the quality categories:

Table 17.2. Performance year (PY) target price transitions (%)

	PY1	PY2	PY3	PY4	PY5
Hospital-specific episode data	66.7	66.7	33.3	0	0
Region-specific episode data	33.3	33.3	66.7	100	100

Table 17.3. Composite score measures and weight for Comprehensive Care for Joint Replacement

Composite score measures	Points (max. 20)	Weight (%)
Hospital-level risk-standardized complication rate following elective primary total hip arthroplasty (THA) and/or total knee arthroplasty (TKA)	10	50
Hospital Consumer Assessment of Health Care Providers and Systems Survey	8	40
THA/TKA voluntary patient-reported outcomes data	2	10

Quality performance points: hip and knee risk-standardized complication rate

Quality improvement points: HCAHPS score

Composite quality score: voluntary submission of above two outcomes

The composite quality score assigns different weights to each of the measures. The measure weights for the composite quality score outlined in table 17.3 are on a publicly reported schedule for both complications and HCAHPS. The patient-reported outcomes measure is a voluntary measure that allows hospital participants to gather important information from patients during pre- and post-anchor discharge. CMS hopes to glean new insights from the patient-reported outcomes measure and test whether this type of measure should be tied to payment in future bundled payment models.

The discount factor also depends on your quality performance within the CJR model. This composite score determines a hospital's eligibility for reconciliation payment and could reduce the 3% discount required by CMS, allowing for an increase in positive reconciliation payment.

The composite score falls into four categories—below acceptable, acceptable, good, and excellent—and affects the discount rate and overall eligibility for reconciliation, as seen in table 17.4.

Table 17.4. Quality categories within Comprehensive Care for Joint Replacement

Year 1	Composite score	Discount factor (%)	Eligible for reconciliation
Below acceptable	Less than 4.0	3.0	No
Acceptable	4.0 to less than 6.0	3.0	Yes
Good	6.0 to less than 13.2	2.0[a]	Yes
Excellent	Above 13.2	1.5[a]	Yes

[a]Discount factor lowered due to quality incentive payment.

As is the theme with many bundled payment models, the largest opportunity for savings (typically 50% of the total opportunity) within Comprehensive Care for Joint Replacement is in the post-acute care space. Employing the concept of care navigators/managers and involving physicians early and often to help you manage and stay close to the patient across the care continuum are a few keys to success within CJR.

Bundled Payment for Care Improvement Advanced

BPCI Advanced builds upon the experience gained on current and previous CMS models and programs, such as the original BPCI, CJR and OCM. Designed around four major facets—payment and risk track election, inpatient clinical episodes, outpatient clinical episodes (new), and target prices—this particular model rewards you if you can deliver high quality care while lowering costs of services provided during the episode of care.

The first group of participants in BPCI Advanced started their participation on October 1, 2018. A second application period will be available for hospitals and physician groups to initiate episodes starting January 1, 2020. The BPCI Advanced model will run in total for five years (beginning from original start date of October 2018) and end on December 31, 2023 for both applicant groups. The model is designed to put the quality of care and health of patients first. It is open to both acute care hospitals and physician group practices. There are also two types of episode initiators within BPCI Advanced:

Conveners: the type of participant that brings together multiple downstream entities, (referred to as episode initiators) and facilitates coordination among them. It bears and apportions financial risk under the model.

Non-conveners: any participant that is itself an episode initiator and bears financial risk only for itself. It does not bear risk on behalf of multiple downstream episode initiators.

BPCI Advanced is a retrospective model that qualifies as an advanced alternative payment model under the Quality Payment Program. The model provides you preliminary pricing targets in advance of each performance period within the model. Your performance will also be tied to quality measures. The program consists of 32 clinical episodes: 29 inpatient and 3 outpatient. The episodes are triggered by the inpatient stay or outpatient procedure. They include the 90-day period starting the day of discharge (see figure 17.1). The episodes combine Medicare-allowed amounts (e.g., fee schedule amounts) as payments for physician, hospital, and other care providers into a single, bundled amount. Your total payments (really, allowed amounts) across services, equipment, and other items provided over a 90-day episode of care are the total episode costs.

A few notable differences with BPCI Advanced compared to the other current models start with precedence rules at the provider level (i.e., attending physician, operating physician, and then the hospital) and at the model or interaction level:

- BPCI Advanced does not have time-based precedence.
- Original BPCI has precedence over CJR.
- CJR has precedence over BPCI Advanced.
- BPCI Advanced episodes will run concurrently with OCM episodes.

Also, reconciliation is semiannual, like that of the OCM (BPCI is quarterly; CJR is annually). The first performance year is immediately at risk (whereas the other models had phased-in risk), and CJR will always take precedence over BPCI Advanced no matter what episode started first.

Bundled Payment Market Dynamics

Existing Bundled Payment Models' Effects on Accountable Care Organizations

Bundled payment and population health programs have been increasing in popularity over the past few years. The Centers for Medicare and Medicaid Services encourages (or mandates, in the case of some CJR markets) participation in bundled payment and other CMS shared savings initiatives, such as ACOs. Beneficiaries can fall into both programs. CMS has defined policies for overlap between these two models, but these policies differ depending on the bundled payment model in question and have been the target of controversy since the BPCI program first started.

As discussed in previous chapters, CMS ACO models promote value at the highest level, with accountability for population cost, quality, and experience over multiple years. CMS ACO models were designed to hold ACOs accountable for the total cost of care of the Medicare beneficiaries aligned with them, regardless of where care is "initiated." Overlap policies have the potential to remove accountability from the ACO for the cost of care during an episode while still holding the ACO accountable for patient experience and quality, thus delinking the components of the Triple Aim (15).

In the original BPCI program, for example, CMS would, for each BPCI awardee or episode initiator that is or is not affiliated with an ACO participant, perform a recoupment calculation for all beneficiaries aligned with that ACO that experienced a BPCI episode during the ACO's performance year. For Comprehensive Care for Joint Replacement, CMS attributes savings achieved during an episode to the CJR participant, and it will include CJR reconciliation payments for ACO-assigned beneficiaries as ACO expenditures.

In the new BPCI Advanced program, CMS will exclude from bundled payment episodes beneficiaries aligned with certain ACOs (Next Generation ACO, prospective Medicare Shared Savings Program [MSSP] Track 3). For other ACOs (MSSP Tracks 1 and 2), the savings attributed to the bundled payment model will be added to ACO expenditures when the beneficiary is ACO-aligned.

While still somewhat a moving target, the overarching goal is that ACOs and bundled payment participants will foster coordination of care and medical information sharing for the patients they serve.

Executing Bundles within an Accountable Care Organization

As you might expect, population health strategies should and can complement each other. These multiple population health strategies should enable you to drive additional savings while achieving economies of scale. On this notion, you can also experiment with implementing the concept of bundled payments directly within an ACO. Your various population health and clinical care teams should not be siloed but instead fully integrated, collaborative, and aligned in both their capabilities and management. This allows you to maximize synergies and economies of scale among your care teams. Simultaneously. You should achieve better outcomes for both your bundled payment program and ACO. In addition, by executing a bundled payment structure inside an ACO, you can engage your specialist physicians by focusing on the management of specific inpatient episodic care (e.g., high-cost/high-opportunity service lines). Bundled payments are a way for ACOs to extend their population health management work to specialists and post-acute providers. You can use nationally recognized bundled payment models as a blueprint. If you already have an established population health infrastructure and access to claims data through the ACO, you can define the episodes ripe for bundle "design." Center your efforts on either chronic disease or surgical episodes. Customize incentives and distribution of gains. You can do all this without the risk associated with formal bundled payment participation.

ACOs operate under a simple premise: through a network of integrated providers and leveraging basic financial incentives, physicians will work together to reduce cost, improve quality, and enhance the health of a set, attributed population. While simple to state, achieving these aims is uniquely difficult. Many ACOs have achieved success working with primary care providers to improve upon preventive health engagement, post-acute provider management, and proactive admission prevention. While these efforts have been fruitful, they have not entirely addressed two key areas: physician–specialist engagement and episodic management.

Using nationally recognized bundled payment models as a blueprint, a bundled payment structure within an ACO program creates cross-continuum (e.g., 90-, 180-day) episodes of care centered on specific disease or procedure groups. By following the bundled payment capabilities outlined later in this chapter, you can realize significant benefits to your ACO. Specifically, specialists would have the opportunity to earn shared savings by achieving quality improvements and reducing the average cost of the bundles compared to the ACO's historical benchmark. As a caveat, the recent rules for both Next Generation and Track 3 ACOs do state that implementing these changes can align specialists, improve episodic care, enhance total shared savings, diversify resources to focus on multiple areas of opportunity, and increase patient, physician, and provider satisfaction.

Although there are numerous benefits to executing this strategy, there are important considerations to examine before implementing this model.

> *Opportunity identification:* Is there enough opportunity? What episodes make the most sense? Where does the most opportunity lie (inpatient and/or post-acute and with which physicians)?
>
> *Specialist engagement and responsibility:* What is the feasibility of engaging and obtaining buy-in or interest from employed or community specialists?
>
> *ACO life cycle:* How new is the ACO? Is there a history of shared savings or not?
>
> *Exclusions:* Within the MSSP Track 3, prospectively assigned beneficiaries are excluded from BPCI Advanced entirely.

Also note that a hospital or physician group who initiates bundled payments but are also part of the ACO may still participate in BPCI Advanced.

Commercial Payers

Because the number of bundle programs are growing, commercial payers are also gaining momentum with their promotion of bundled payments. Large commercial payers and some large employers are signing bundled payment contracts for specific conditions. For example, Horizon Blue Cross Blue Shield of New Jersey announced successful outcomes from its Episodes of Care program (16). Horizon reviewed its 2014 claims data for members receiving care from practices participating in this program and compared the results with patients receiving care for the same procedures from nonparticipating practices. Outcomes demonstrated 100% fewer hospital readmissions for knee arthroscopy, 37% fewer readmissions for hip replacements, 22% fewer readmissions for knee replacements, and a 32% reduction in unnecessary caesarian sections.

There are significant differences in the opportunities for cost reduction depending on the acute care episode, geography, and the patient population (i.e., commercial vs. Medicare). According to recent studies, admissions and post-acute care are responsible for a relatively small percentage of the average total–bundled payment for total knee and hip joint surgery for commercial patients as compared to Medicare patients. For example, the variability in utilization of commercial patients residing in the Mountain region discharged to self-care at home ranged from 59% as compared to only 18% in the New England region. In addition, the commercial bundled cost differences in geographic regions for those patients accessing post-acute care services range from $3,907 to $5,292: a difference of nearly $1,400 (17).

These are critical factors to consider when selecting payers and acute care episodes. Additional topics essential for getting started with the commercial bundled payment agreements include, but are not limited to, the following:

- Current volume of patients in the proposed bundle with the payer
- Ability to evaluate payer claims for utilization and costs for *all* services in the bundle

- Payer's ability to modify its claims processing methodologies
- Sensitivity stress test of the relationship between operational and clinical efficiencies and financial performance. The test should identify the primary drivers of risk within the bundled payment business model, and scenarios can include assessing the impact of post-acute care utilization, not achieving the desired length of stay and/or supply cost reduction targets, increases in related emergency department visits or readmissions, and negative shifts in market share.
- An evaluation of adequate stop-loss provisions is key to provide protection against outliers.
- Essential components of a communication and marketing plan
- Benefit design incentives to include, over time, an increase in volume as a preferred provider from the payer

Bundled payment programs with commercial payers or employers can benefit all parties involved:

- Patients may benefit from reduced variability, better quality, clear expectations of the pathway, better communication across the continuum of care with providers, and less out-of-pocket expenses.
- Hospitals, health systems, and physicians may find that although the volume of services within the episode is reduced, the overall volume of episodes increases through preferred provider status. In addition, as a result of participation in these programs, providers may develop capabilities essential to success with the introduction of other alternative payment models.
- Physicians and other patient care providers may benefit from better alignment of the provision of care and related responsibilities across the continuum that is prompted by the bundled payment program.
- Physicians and other patient care providers may also benefit from separate gain-sharing agreements with the provider. The agreements would reward high-quality care delivered with improved cost efficiency.

- Commercial payers will benefit from a discounted fee arrangement and the chance to partner with a provider willing to work to improve care delivery to the payer's beneficiaries.

Core Capabilities Needed for Success in Bundled Payment
Leadership, Governance, and Infrastructure

You should have a governance structure that provides oversight and support for the bundled payment program and the various work streams associated with transforming care delivery. Before diving into the nuts and bolts of program design, strong executive sponsorship and the commitment of physician/clinical champions are essential. Organizations that show positive outcomes and cost savings develop aligned goals for their bundled payment initiatives. They invest in structure and resources designed to facilitate high performance within an episode of care. One layer down, leadership generally creates a multidisciplinary oversight or steering committee to manage the day-to-day work and optimize performance. Successful bundled payment models need to be one of your core strategic goals for the organization. If treated as such, the organization will garner savings (i.e., increased revenue opportunities). Bundled payment programs are not isolated projects.

Model and Episode Design Knowledge

Whether a Medicare-sponsored bundle or a commercial or employer bundle contract, having a point person who understands the details about the program is essential. This includes an overall understanding of the operational processes and practices of the organization, as well as knowledge of bundled payment program elements: how to define the bundle and determine the target price, how to negotiate or manage the overall stop-gain/stop-loss cap, and how to describe the impact on overall volume of beneficiary inclusions/exclusions. Also important is for you to identify someone who understands program precedence, reconciliation rules, and repayment practices. This individual or individuals should be part of the steering committee and help inform that group's activities.

Targeted Analytics and Episode Selection

Your ability to measure, monitor, and evaluate current bundle performance, as well as forecast for the future, is critical for sustaining a bundled payment program. Detailed claims and eligibility data is complex, but also a very rich resource for providing detailed information across the care continuum (inpatient, professional visits, and post-acute care). Claims analytics capabilities—as well as the ability to enhance an electronic medical record for patient tracking, clinical protocols and order sets, and the ability to provide data to key stakeholders (e.g., surgeons, physicians)—is critical.

A well-structured bundled payment program could still be financially unsuccessful. Lack of success occurs when the episodes selected don't have a strong savings opportunity and the providers involved don't have an ability to influence change. To begin, leadership needs to collect and analyze financial and clinical data to determine those episodes that have the widest variation in terms of cost and quality. Such situations represent the greatest opportunities for savings. Most successful choices tend to be episodes with significant overutilization of post-acute care. Additionally, high-volume, high-dollar procedures that rely on expensive resources (such as physician preference items like implants that range widely in cost) have variable outcomes in terms of quality (such as higher than expected complications). The addition of higher readmission rates leads to much higher costs. Similarly, the providers in the bundle have to have an influence over the cost and quality outcomes. Episode choices are most successful when there are preexisting evidence-based quality and efficiency metrics that align with the program goal. Additionally, procedures can be easily modified to reflect the most appropriate needs of the patient as they move to the next step in their care journey (e.g., post-discharge/procedure).

Cross-Continuum Care Delivery and Management— Clinical Transformation

Due to the cross-continuum nature of bundles, your ability to assess and redesign care across the episode (i.e., find and close care gaps) and to execute continuous improvement processes to achieve both low-cost and high-quality outcomes is another core program capability. Historically, providers have been narrowly focused on the procedures or interventions that will be done in the acute care setting, along with the immediate preoperative and postoperative care. However, organizations successful in bundles have invested in care management and patient navigators that can develop a plan for prehospitalization care all the way through the post-discharge period (e.g. 90 days), which coordinates handoffs between providers and minimizes use of more expensive resources. For example, your care plan may involve utilizing home health or outpatient care to avoid placement in a skilled nursing facility that can often cost four times as much. Alternatively, you can educate the patient and family on exactly when (and when not) to present to the emergency room for care.

Procedural and chronic bundles have different care coordination challenges. Focusing on patient optimization, coordination, and communication with primary care and leveraging community resources are common care delivery approaches.

Patient Engagement and Protections

You should be intentional about establishing a patient notification process (e.g., start of episode) and introduce the care team early on in the episode of care. Provide a customized patient and family education process and needs assessment during both the hospital stay and throughout post-acute care phase (18). Your ability to protect patients from unintended underutilization of appropriate services both ensures better outcomes and encourages compliance with care plans (19).

Post-Acute Care

Post-acute care is perhaps the most significant contributor toward your total per episode spending for many episodes of care (20). For example, post-acute care and readmissions account for nearly 40% of Medicare spending for 30-day heart failure episodes and 37% of spending for joint replacement episodes (3). Therefore, developing a preferred and narrow network of high-quality, low-cost post-acute care providers is an essential component of success in bundled payment. An evaluative process is suggested to strategically identify and select partners for preferred designation. Leverage on-site assessments (e.g., not just a handpicked reports) of post-acute providers, as well as public data sets. Consider star ratings, readmission rates, patient satisfaction scores, and so on to ensure only those with demonstrable cost and quality outcomes are selected for inclusion. Partners must also be willing to agree upon and adopt practice tools and processes that standardize patient experience and promote quality outcomes. Note that not all post-acute providers offer high-quality across all bundles. Therefore, the inclusion of satisfaction scores, along with other quality criteria, can better ensure only those with demonstrable cost and quality outcomes are selected. Your partners must also be willing to agree upon and adopt practice tools and processes that standardize the patient experience and promote quality outcomes. Therefore, there may be different designated networks depending on the patient's needs.

Provider Alignment

Provider alignment and engagement typically involves a two-pronged approach. One is based on structures that promote transparency and continual communication. The other is founded on incentives to influence behavior change. Your engagement structures need to allow physicians and other leaders to meet regularly on shared discussion topics, such as progress to goals, quality, redesign efforts, data sharing, and data transparency.

In addition, your providers need to use established communication channels, such as clinician-champion communication trees, provider meetings, newsletters, emails, one-on-one discussions, and so on. These channels will inform and disclose information among participants. Additionally, new communication channels may be added to supplement those already existing. Providing support for clinical champions with project management, change management, and leadership training is also crucial yet often undervalued.

Alignment structures often come in the form of incentives contingent upon hitting quality and outcomes goals and savings achieved. By choosing your performance measures and corresponding targets carefully, hospitals and physicians can find themselves in a win-win scenario with better compensation tied to improved patient outcomes delivered at a lower cost. Key strategies include consideration of both financial and nonfinancial incentives for physicians, such as increased transparency of outcomes across the continuum, improved patient access to appropriate providers, advanced alternative payment model qualification, and exploration (or development) of gain-sharing opportunities.

Summary

Bundled payments represent a key strategy for you to explore on the journey toward value-based care. Especially consider how each of the bundled payment capabilities and strategies outlined in this chapter can directly cross-pollinate into the work within an ACO structure. There are more synergies than you think that can be leveraged across teams in both programs. Bundled payment models have been in operation for decades though on a much more limited scale than we see today. Numerous tests of change have shown that these models can be leveraged to generate both cost and quality improvements for a range of clinical episodes. Bundled payments can also help providers accelerate their movement toward risk-based contracting while allowing time to optimize performance before building advanced capabilities.

In addition, bundled payments can help you yield significant margin opportunities from your health system. Bundling offers the chance to earn over 50% of all Medicare savings if successful. However, not everyone achieves success.

To build a successful program, providers need to commit to change. They must recruit partners and participants that are willing to take the journey toward continuous performance improvement. Leadership must support the effort with a true commitment of time and resources. Leadership needs to provide management structures and infrastructures to oversee the program and monitor performance. Episodes must be carefully selected based on data, provider, and market analysis to uncover the greatest areas of opportunity. Care design must be considered all along the continuum to ensure optimal performance. Lastly, incentives need to be managed to encourage the right behaviors at the right pace of change.

If you can home in on the capabilities outlined in this chapter and attain successful collaboration with your care teams and hospital leadership, you will start seeing accelerated performance improvement within your bundled payment programs.

REFERENCES

1. Shih T, Chen LM, Nallamothu BK. Will bundled payments change health care? Examining the evidence thus far in cardiovascular care. *Circulation.* 2015;131(24):2151–2158.

2. Conrad DA. The theory of value-based payment incentives and their application to health care. *Health Serv Res.* 2015;50(Suppl 2):2057–2089. doi:10.1111/1475-6773.12408.

3. Mechanic R. *Medicare's Bundled Payment Initiatives: Considerations for Providers.* Washington, DC: American Hospital Association; 2016. https://www.aha.org/system/files/content/16/issbrief-bundledpmt.pdf. Accessed October 23, 2019.

4. Comprehensive care for joint replacement model. Centers for Medicare and Medicaid Services website. https://innovation.cms.gov/initiatives/cjr. Accessed October 23, 2019.

5. Oncology care model. Centers for Medicare and Medicaid Services website. https://innovation.cms.gov/initiatives/oncology-care. Accessed October 23, 2019.

6. Lewin Group. *CMS Bundled Payments for Care Improvement Initiative Models 2-4: Year 3 Evaluation and Monitoring Annual Report.* Falls Church, VA: Lewin Group; 2017. https://downloads.cms.gov/files/cmmi/bpci-models2-4yr3evalrpt.pdf. Updated October 2018. Accessed October 23, 2019.

7. Premier Inc. CJR participants outperform peers in achieving savings by 35% [press release]. Charlotte, NC: Premier Inc.; November 20, 2017. https://www.premierinc.com/premier-inc-cjr-participants-outperform-peers-achieving-savings-35/. Accessed October 23, 2019.

8. PWC. *2015/2016 Results: Hospitals, Employers, and Consumers Survey.* https://www.strategyand.pwc.com/media/file/Annual-Bundles-Survey-2015-2016-Results.pdf Accessed October 23, 2019.

9. Where commercial and employer bundled payments stand in healthcare right now. *Becker's Hospital CFO Report.* June 27, 2013. https://www.beckershospitalreview.com/finance/where-commercial-and-employer-bundled-payments-stand-in-healthcare-right-now.html. Accessed October 23, 2019.

10. Mouille B, Higuera C, Woicehovich L, Deadwiler, M. How to succeed in bundled payments for joint replacement [case study]. *NEJM Catalyst.* October 24, 2016. https://catalyst.nejm.org/how-to-succeed-in-bundled-payments-for-total-joint-replacement. Accessed October 23, 2019.

11. Miller DC, Gust C, Dimick JB, Birkmeyer N, Skinner J, Birkmeyer JD. Large variations in Medicare payments for surgery highlight savings potential from bundled payment programs. *Health Aff (Millwood)*. 2011;30(11):2107-2105. doi:10.1377/hlthaff.2011.0783.

12. Oncology care model [fact sheet]. *CMS.gov Newsroom*. June 29, 2016. https://www.cms.gov/newsroom/fact-sheets/oncology-care-model. Accessed October 23, 2019.

13. American Cancer Society. *Cancer Facts & Figures 2016*. Atlanta, GA: American Cancer Society; 2016. http://www.cancer.org/research/cancerfactsstatistics /cancerfactsfigures2016/index. Accessed May 22, 2018.

14. Ellison A. Proposed changes to CJR model will cost Medicare $90M over next 3 years. *Becker's Hospital CFO Report*. October 11, 2017. https://www .beckershospitalreview.com/finance/proposed-changes-to-cjr-model-will-cost -medicare-90m-over-next-3-years.html. Accessed May 22, 2018.

15. Letter to CMS voicing concerns about overlap of bundles and ACOs. National Association of ACOs website. April 26, 2016. https://www.naacos.com /letter-to-cms-voicing-concerns-about-overlap-of-bundles-and-acos. Accessed October 23, 2019.

16. Horizon BCBSNJ members all win from company's innovative "Episodes of Care" program [press release]. Blue Cross Blue Shield website. February 17, 2016. https://www.bcbs.com/news/press-releases/horizon-bcbsnj-members-all-win-companys -innovative-episodes-care-program. Accessed May 15, 2018.

17. Bundled pricing for total joint replacements in the commercially insured population: geographic variation and cost-driver insights [research brief]. Truven Health Analytics; January 2016. Accessed May 10, 2018.

18. Bernabeo E, Holmboe ES. Patients, providers, and systems need to acquire a specific set of competencies to achieve truly patient-centered care. *Health Aff (Millwood)*. 2013;32(2):250–258. doi:10.1377/hlthaff.2012.1120.

19. Carman KL, Dardess P, Maurer M, et al. Patient and family engagement: a framework for understanding the elements and developing interventions and policies. *Health Aff (Millwood)*. 2013;32(2):223–231. doi:10.1377/hlthaff.2012.1133.

20. Gosfield A. Bundled payment: avoiding surprise packages. In: Gosfield A, ed. *Health Law Handbook*. 25th ed. Eagan, MN: Westlaw; 2013.

Afterword

Medicare has decided to alter the payment system because of the perception of too many perverse incentives. In 2015, Congress passed the MACRA (Medicare Access and CHIP Reauthorization Act) legislation to attempt to deal with this issue.

A critical part of the MACRA legislation was to create a quality improvement incentive called MIPS (Merit-based Incentive Payment System). MIPS combines the old Physician Quality Reporting System, Value-Based Payment Modifier, and Medicare EHR Incentive Program. Understanding the difference between APM (Alternative Payment Model) and Advanced APM will be critical to success with the program.

There are strict rules for determining who is a Qualified Physician (QP). Under MIPS there are four performance categories you will need to complete:

1. Quality
2. Promoting Interoperability (formerly Advancing Care Information)
3. Cost
4. Clinical Practice Improvement Activities

These are complicated scoring methods.

To understand all of this better, refer to the 2019 edition of *The ACO Guide to MACRA* (https://Naacos.memberclicks.net/assets/docs/pdf/macra /TheACO_GuidetoMACRA_2019EditionFullReport022019v2.pdf).

Page numbers in *italics* refer to figures and tables.

commercial payers: bundled payment programs and, 302–4; two-sided risk arrangements and, 143, 144–45

communication: about QMV audits, 120; about two-sided risk models, 154–55; in bundled payment programs, 307; care coordination and, 85–87, 86, 88

compensation, criteria for, 26, 154

competition: differentiation from, and bundled payment programs, 287–88; for medical talent, 150; opportunities for two-sided risk and, 150–53

compliance considerations, 213, 217–19

Comprehensive Care for Joint Replacement (CJR), 284, 285, 293–97, 295, 296, 297

Comprehensive Primary Care Initiative (CPCI), 271–72

Comprehensive Primary Care Payment, 277

Comprehensive Primary Care Plus (CPC+) program: attribution methodology of, 275; drivers of, 273, 274; dual participation in ACO model and, 279–81; as multi-payer approach, 277–78; as option for ACOs, 28–29; overview of, 271–72; participation in, 272–73; payment innovations of, 276–77; Quality Payment Program and, 278–79; quality reporting requirements for, 278; shared savings opportunities and, 263; tiered approach of, 274–75

continuously assigned patient population, 209–11

contracts: attribution and, 196; commercial, for Optimus Healthcare Partners, 256–57; with data analytics vendors, 193–95; as portfolios of risk relationships, 202

COPD (chronic obstructive pulmonary disease), 248–49

costs: of health care, 91, 222; of MSSP, 114–15; of post-acute care, 165–67, 166, 167

cost savings: distribution and history of, 19–20; of Hackensack Alliance ACO, 20, 21, 22

CPC+. See Comprehensive Primary Care Plus Program

CPCI (Comprehensive Primary Care Initiative), 271–72

Crossing the Quality Chasm (Institute of Medicine), 38, 93

culture: high-value, 24; of PCMHs, 50–53; in wellness and prevention programs, 233

data analysis / data analytics: attribution and, 195–96; for bundled payment programs, 305; for care coordination, 62; claim and claim line feeds and, 10; contracts for outside-sourced information and, 193–95; for employee health plan management, 227–29; evolution of capabilities in, 196–97; external financial and quality reporting and, 197–98; NQF and, xiv; overview of, 191–92, 201–2; payer-based analytics, 198–99; in practice transformation, 259–60; purpose of, 191; risk adjustment and, 201; in selection of post-acute partners, 181–82; vendors of, 192–93

data management in two-sided risk contracts, 157–58

delivery of primary care, 243–45

determinants of health, xiv–xv

diagnosis codes, 245

diagnosis-related groups, xii, 2, 25, 209, 285–86

direct-to-employer agreements with health care provider organizations, 225–26, 236, 236–37, 263

discharge planning and post-acute referrals, 179

disease management in employee health plans, 231–32

disincentives for high-cost care settings, 230–31

distribution of net savings to providers, 19–20, 260

documentation: for care coordination, 63–64, 69–70, 82–83; error categories in, 123–25; for PCMHs, 44–50; QMV audits of, 117–18, 133–36; risk scoring and, 203–4, 205, 206

100; EHR API Connector, 104, 106, 108–9; gap analysis tool of, 105, 106; GPRO survey and, 119; optimal gaps tool of, 110–11; patient assignment algorithm of, 104, 104; Provider Performance Scorecards, 107, 109; role of, 10; secure text message notifications of, 106, 107; submissions to WI and, 101–2

Health Enhancement Research Organization, 224

health maintenance organizations (HMOs), xi, 2, 240

health savings accounts, 230

healthy living, incentives for, 230

Henry Ford Health System, 226

hierarchical condition categories/codes (HCCs), 144, 204–6, 205, 207–8, 209–10

high-cost care settings, disincentives for, 230–31

high-deductible health plans, 230

Hippocrates of Kos, x

HMOs (health maintenance organizations), xi, 2, 240

home health agencies: hospital-owned, 177; post-acute care by, 161, 163, 165

Horizon Blue Cross Blue Shield of New Jersey, 254, 257, 302

Hospital Consumer Assessment of Healthcare Providers and Systems (HCAHPS), 295–96

hospitalists, 67

hospitalizations: reducing, 35; tracking, 49, 62; transitions from, 67, 80–81; waste, misdirected care, and, 248–49

Improving Medicare Post-Acute Care Transformation (IMPACT) Act of 2014, 163–65, 164

incentives: bundled payment programs and, 283, 285–87, 308; in contracts, 193–94; under diagnosis-related groups, 25; in health care financing model, 247–48; for healthy living and preventative care, 230; for performance improvement, 259, 260–62; perverse, 311; for physician engagement, 36–37, 154; in post-acute care,

68, 160, 164; in provider networks, 235–36. See also alternative payment models; Medicare Shared Savings Program; Merit-based Incentive Payment System

independent physician associations (IPAs), 253–54

infrastructure duplication, 146

inpatient rehabilitation facilities and post-acute care, 162, 164, 165

Institute of Medicine: Care Management Plan, 291, 291; Crossing the Quality Chasm, 38, 93; To Err Is Human, 92

insurers, negotiation of change with, 249–51

integrated health care systems, physician practice groups as, 253

IPAs (independent physician associations), 253–54

Jenner, Edward, x

Johnson, Lyndon, xi

Joint Commission, The: Codman and creation of, xii; PCMHs and, 23, 40, 53–55, 54

joint operating arrangements, 171

joint operating committees or collaboratives, 171, 173–74

joint ownerships in post-acute care, 172, 172–73

joint replacement bundled payment program, 250, 284, 293–97, 295, 296, 297

joint ventures: in employee health plan management, 222; in post-acute care, 171, 172, 172–73

Kerth, Norman, 132–33

Koch, Robert, xi

leadership: of bundled payment programs, 304; of networks, 185; by PCPs, 242; by physician champions, 255–56, 259; two-sided risk models and, 154–55; wellness and prevention programs and, 233

legal considerations, 213–17

Lister, Joseph, x

lists, high-risk, 68–69

population health management
consulting: benchmarking performance data and, 270; need for,
265–67, 266; overview of, 264, 270;
plan for and speed of transition and,
267, 267–70
post-acute care (PAC): ACOs and,
165–67; alignment with providers of,
168; building and managing networks
with, 185–86; bundled payments and,
286–87, 306–7; care coordinators
and, 68; clinical transformation and,
186–88; cost of, 165–67, 166, 167;
definition of, 160–61; driving quality
in, 188–90; elements of success in,
190; engagement and collaboration
with, 169–76, 171, 178–80; home
health agencies and, 161; in inpatient
rehabilitation facilities, 162; in
long-term acute care hospitals, 162;
monitoring, 25; ownership of assets
for, 171, 172–73, 176–78; partnering
with providers of, 160, 181–84;
payment and reimbursement for,
163–64, 164; quality of, 164–65; in
SNFs, 161–62; in two-sided risk
contracts, 156
post-discharge home visit waivers, 216
preferred provider networks, 174–76,
175, 235–36
preferred provider organizations (PPOs),
xi–xii
Premier Inc., 10, 22, 145, 151, 221
premiums, amount of, 250
pre-participation waivers, 215
preventative care, incentives for, 230
primary care attribution process, 152,
195–96
primary care physicians/providers
(PCPs): assignment of, 47, 104, 104;
definition of, 17; delivery of care by,
243–45; evolution of, 239–40;
expansion of providers of, 242–43;
leadership of ACOs by, 242; medication management and, 247;
overview of, 252; patient-provider
relationships in, 251–52; role of,
241–42; services provided by, 245–46;
team-based care and, 246–47

Privia, 145
productivity of care coordination, 72–73
*Project Retrospectives: A Handbook for
Team Reviews* (Kerth), 132–33
prospective beneficiary assignment, 195
provider agreements, 184
provider participation criteria for
networks, 156
PwC Health Research Institute, 225–26

QMV audits. *See* quality measure
validation (QMV) audits
qualified participants (QPs), 27–28
Qualified Physicians (QPs), 311
quality domains and quality scores,
115
quality improvement process, 97–98
quality measures/metrics: in bundled
payment programs, 289; collecting,
scoring, and reporting, 100; for CPC+,
278; evolution of, xii–xv; focus on,
92–93; health care organizations as
driving, 251; in measure sets, 95,
95–96; for Oncology Care Model,
292; oversight of, 94–95; overview of,
91–92; in post-acute care, 188–90; in
success of ACOs, 98–99; for Web
Interface, 100–101
quality measure validation (QMV)
audits: analysis and results of,
121–25, 122; documentation
collection and submission for, 133–36;
methodology for, 118–19, 119;
mismatch detail, 136–41; mismatch
error categories in, 123–25; need for,
115–16; notification of, 119–20;
objectives of, 116; overview of,
112–13; recommendations for,
131–33; response to, 125–31; scope
of, 117–18; steps in response to,
120–21
quality of care: evolution of assessment
of, xii–xv; in post-acute care, 164–65,
188–90; in SNFs, 165. *See also* quality
measures; quality measure validation
(QMV) audits
quality outcomes: for care coordination, 70–72; PCMHs and, 35–36,
49–50

teams: for care coordination, 61–63, 66, 73, 89; for PCMHs, 45–46; for primary care, 246–47; for QMV audits, 120, 125, 132. *See also* Comprehensive Primary Care Plus (CPC+) program

technology and care management systems, 157. *See also* electronic medical record (EMR) systems

telehealth originating site waivers, 216

telemedicine, 243

Telligen, 120

templates for care coordination documentation, 69–70

third-party administrators (TPAs), 228–29, 232

To Err Is Human (Institute of Medicine), 92

Track 1: application to, 4; as learning laboratory, 269–70; overview of, 5, 142; risk and, 6; unavailability of, 8

Track 1+, 4, 5, 6, 147, 148

Track 2, 4, 5, 6

Track 3, 4, 5, 6, 301

training: of advanced nurse practitioners, 242–43; in care coordination, 66, 75, 86; in response to QMV audits, 128; in workflow, 105

transformation of practices: bundled payments and, 287, 305–6; to CPC+, 274–75; as long-term process, 27; to PCMHs, 44; post-acute care and, 186–88. *See also* Optimus Healthcare Partners; population health management consulting

transitional contacts, 67, 80–81

transition assistants, 71

transparency: of Hackensack Alliance, 1; in QMV audits, 120, 132; of results, as goal of MSSP, 9

"tribal knowledge" about post-acute care, overcoming, 177, 180

Triple Aim, ix, xiii, 9

"2 plus 1" staffing model for PCMHs, 43

two-sided risk arrangements: CJR as, 293; factors in success of, 153–58; growth in, 144–45; with guardrails, 147; market dynamics and, 150–53; negotiations for terms of, 147–48, 155; overview of, 145–46, 147, 158–59; in Pathways to Success, 149; payment waivers in, 214. *See also* Advanced Alternative Payment Model; alternative payment models

types or forms of ACOs, 4

UnitedHealthcare, 145

upside models, 145

urgent care centers, 34, 244

Utilization Review Accreditation Commission (URAC), 40, 53–55, 54

validation, definition of, 114

value-based payment (VBP) model, 203–6, 212, 260. *See also* bundled payment programs; Comprehensive Primary Care Plus (CPC+) program; Optimus Healthcare Partners; population health management consulting

value of services, assessment of, ix

venture capital-based companies, 152

Vigorita, John, 256

Vista Healthcare System IPA, 253

waivers: available to MSSP models, 217; available under Pathways to Success, 218; compliance requirements for, 217–19; fraud and abuse, 213, 215–16; payment, 214, 215, 216–17; of three-day skilled nursing facility stay rule, 7, 187–88, 216

waste, identification and reduction of, 248–49

Web Interface (WI): MIPS and, 100; quality measures and, 100–101; submissions to, 101–7, 110–11

wellness and prevention programs, 232–33

workflows in care coordination, 78–81, 84–85, 87